CASE STUDIES OF EXCEPTIONAL STUDENTS

Handicapped and Gifted

ABOUT THE AUTHOR

Carroll J. Jones received her Ph.D. in Special Education Administration and Learning Disabilities from Kansas State University and her M.Ed. in Reading and B.A. in Elementary Education from the University of Arizona. Doctor Jones's primary interests are in the areas of teacher training at small colleges, mildly handicapped students, and the social and emotional development of handicapped students. As an Associate Professor at Lander College, Doctor Jones was instrumental in designing one of the first B.S. degree programs in South Carolina for training teachers of mildly handicapped students. At the Associated Colleges of Central Kansas, she implemented the first undergraduate teacher training program in learning disabilities in Kansas. While at Fayetteville State University, North Carolina, Doctor Jones served as a training consultant on a federal Special Education Consultation Grant to imbed collaborative consultation training into a Master's Degree program in Special Education.

Currently, Doctor Jones is on professional sabbatical in Germany, writing books about the social and self-concept aspects of educating handicapped students and completing a series of books on teaching mildly handicapped students.

CASE STUDIES OF EXCEPTIONAL STUDENTS

Handicapped and Gifted

By

CARROLL J. JONES, PH.D.

CHARLES C THOMAS • PUBLISHER

Springfield • Illinois • U.S.A.

Published and Distributed Throughout the World by

CHARLES C THOMAS • PUBLISHER
2600 South First Street
Springfield, Illinois 62794-9265

ISBN 0-398-05856-3

Library of Congress Catalog Card Number: 93-6745

With THOMAS BOOKS *careful attention is given to all details of manufacturing and design. It is the Publisher's desire to present books that are satisfactory as to their physical qualities and artistic possibilities and appropriate for their particular use.* THOMAS BOOKS *will be true to those laws of quality that assure a good name and good will.*

Printed in the United States of America
SC-R-3

Library of Congress Cataloging-in-Publication Data

Jones, Carroll J.
Case studies of exceptional students : handicapped and gifted / by Carroll J. Jones.
p. cm.
Includes bibliographical references (p.) and index.
ISBN 0-398-05856-3
1. Exceptional children—Education—United States—Case studies.
2. Handicapped children—Education—United States—Case studies.
3. Gifted children—Education—United States—Case studies.
I. Title.
LC3981.J66 1993
371.9'0973—dc20 93-6745
CIP

To Andrea and Camille,
Martha and Rachael

FOREWORD

Teacher training programs in both special and regular education have a large body of information at the knowledge level for acquisition by prospective teachers. Having a solid knowledge base about what to do with exceptional students in the regular or special education classroom is important, but only a small part of the victory in teacher training. Knowing how to and actually applying the knowledge with real students is the real victory. Teacher trainers are constantly discussing, experimenting with, and questioning their efforts at the application level. Few teacher education programs are completely satisfied with the depth and breadth of practical application experiences afforded their pre-service teachers. There is a continuing search for more and better ways to help prospective teachers to have a more realistic idea of the functioning abilities and potential weaknesses of students they may encounter at a variety of ages and with various exceptionalities.

One teaching aid that can provide the basis for a veritable gold mine of practical application experiences about these educationally challenged or gifted students is *Case Studies of Exceptional Students: Handicapped and Gifted.* Dr. Jones is a master at composing, collecting, compiling, and editing clear, concise and educationally relevant case studies helpful for bridging the gap between knowledge about exceptional students and the ability to deal with them in a professionally effective way in the classroom. These case studies (not easily come by for most professors on their own) provide the basis for a myriad of applied activities such as application of identification criteria, Individualized Education Program development and other program planning activities, parent support planning, and preparation of learning style activities. These case studies can greatly lessen the anxieties and unknowns of initial interactions with exceptional students. This is important for potential special educators, but is particularly vital for regular educators who traditionally have less opportunity to acquire a strong knowledge base in special education and even less opportunity to experience in depth practical experiences with these students they may encounter in the mainstream.

Dr. Jones is to be applauded once again for her ability to provide a valuable and versatile teaching supplement which can have so many practical applications in the teacher training program arena. Her broad and deep knowledge of exceptionalities in general and special students in specific has enabled her to provide instructors of introductory and higher level education courses with this useful accompaniment to their texts, periodical resources, and media presentations.

VIRGINIA J. DICKENS, PH.D.
Coordinator, Special Education
Fayetteville State University
Fayetteville, North Carolina

PREFACE

All states require that students in teacher training programs take an introductory course in special education which includes information about special education history and law, and each of the major categories of exceptional students (learning disabled, communication impaired, mentally retarded, severely and multihandicapped, vision impaired, hearing impaired, physically impaired, health impaired, gifted and talented). Introductory special education textbooks typically include one chapter on each of the exceptionalities covering characteristics from birth through adulthood, possible causes, some teaching techniques, and special adaptive equipment.

Most of the students taking these introductory courses are relatively unfamiliar with the characteristics and learning needs of exceptional students, special education acronyms, and education "lingo" that make the linguistic and concept load of an introductory course very heavy. Students frequently experience difficulty understanding special education procedures such as multidisciplinary evaluation, diagnosis, and placement.

A major purpose of this book is to be a companion text to the introduction to special education books currently used by providing case studies of exceptional students with typical profiles to illustrate the generic characteristics and needs of the various exceptionalities. Lists of generic characteristics are difficult to remember, but when they become Megan or Brian or Mark or Diana's handicapping conditions and educational concerns, the characteristics are personalized and more easily understood. Case studies analyzed prior to actual classroom observations will give students in teacher training programs a better idea of the learning characteristics and problems that they will be observing.

Additionally, many special education professors have limited access to case studies of exceptional students due to confidentiality issues. Creating numerous case study reports is not only very time consuming, but may require medical information (e.g., vision diagnosis, physical therapy report) which the average professor teaching introductory courses understands but does not have the background to create. Thus, another major purpose of this text is to provide professors with a readily available set of case studies for students to use in learning about exceptional students.

The case studies in this text are "hypothetical students" with commonly found profiles among exceptional students. Since some states have specific diagnostic characteristics that differ from others (e.g., specific learning disabilities, mildly mentally retarded), there is no attempt to meet those specific requirements, but to provide generic case study examples in each major exceptionality. Some case study students have more than one handicapping condition and, thus, the categories may seem to overlap. This is a realistic situation. However, the text can easily be used in conjunction with individual state eligibility criteria and procedures.

The book is organized into eight chapters including case studies of students ranging from preschool age/grade through secondary age/grade. The chapters focus on specific exceptionalities as follows: Vision Impaired (Chapter One), Communication Impaired (Chapter Two), Hearing Impaired (Chapter Three), Mentally Retarded (Chapter Four), Behavior Disordered (Chapter Five), Learning Disabled (Chapter Six), Physically and Other Health Impaired (Chapter Seven), Gifted (Chapter Eight).

Thanks to my husband who understands that there is "always" a book in process.

This book is dedicated to Andrea and Camille Jones, and Martha and Rachael Dickens, each exceptional in her own special way.

C.J.J.

CONTENTS

CASE STUDIES
OF
EXCEPTIONAL STUDENTS
Handicapped and Gifted

Chapter One

CASES OF VISUALLY IMPAIRED STUDENTS

"Vision impairment is a low-prevalence handicapping condition including children who have never had any visual functioning, those who had normal vision prior to the severe impairment, those who have other handicapping conditions, and those with selective impairments of parts of the visual field. Educators differentiate between blind (reads braille) and low-vision (reads print) students". (Jones, 1992, 43)

Preschool Age/Grade: See Cara
Primary Age/Grade: See Mark
Intermediate Age/Grade: Nicole
  See Also: Heather
Secondary Age/Grade: See Sam & Randy

RE-EVALUATION REPORT
NICOLE

Age: 12 years, 5 months
Grade: 6th Grade
Date: January , 19____

Background and Educational Concerns

Reason for Referral

Nicole is a 12 year, 5 month old 6th grade student attending regular classes at Mitchell Elementary School. Currently, Nicole (who is legally blind) is functioning on grade level using large print books and materials, recorded books, and recorded compressed speech textbook chapters. She uses a computer with oversized monitor and 14 point type to prepare her assignments. There are no social behavioral concerns.

The purpose of this special re-evaluation is to prepare for Nicole's transition to the Junior High School in the fall. Her textbooks and educational materials must be ordered 6 months in advance from the American Printing House of the Blind.

Health

Immunizations are current. Recent physical examination indicated no specific medical concerns.

Vision

Nicole was diagnosed legally blind as an infant. Measured central visual acuity with spectacle correction is 20/200. Eye contact, fixation, and tracking are normal. Fundus examination was normal.

Hearing Screening: Normal Range Auditory Acuity

Speech and Language Screenings

School screenings indicate speech and language functioning are within age expectations. Nicole is verbally spontaneous, has a superior vocabulary, and speaks in grammatically correct sentences.

Behavior

Teachers report that Nicole's social behavior is appropriate for age expectations. Nicole tends to be rather quiet and shy, but is liked by all students in the classroom and spends much of her free time with several girls who have been close friends since kindergarten. On small group projects she is always chosen first due to her good computer skills in report preparation. Nicole becomes frustrated if she is expected to do considerable amount of content reading as it is so much slower than her recorded materials, and the large-print books are so large and bulky to manipulate.

Socio-Economic and Home Information

English is the language of the home. Nicole is the only child of a computer programmer (mother) and computer analyst (father) who own and operate their own very successful business. The family lives in a new ranch style home in a middle-class neighborhood. They maintain a home computer library with numerous computers and a multitude of hardware and software. The parents, not only devised the specific computer apparatus to fulfill Nicole's needs, but set up a complete computer center for her at school as well as at home. They have donated considerable amount of time to the school in establishing the school computer library. Nicole has regular chores about the home. There is no socioeconomic deprivation.

CURRENT MULTIDISCIPLINARY EVALUATION

This evaluation includes intelligence, perception and memory, academic achievement, social skills, and adaptive behavior.

Psychological Evaluation

Test Administered

Wechsler Intelligence Scale for Children-Revised (WISC–R)

Verbal IQ	*120*	Performance IQ (Not administered due to legal blindness)
Information	*14*	
Similarities	*14*	

Arithmetic	*13*
Vocabulary	*12*
Comprehension	*14*
Digit Span	*13*

Test Interpretation

Nicole is a 12 year, 5 month old 6th grade student, who is legally blind, but functioning on grade level in the regular classroom. She entered the testing situation politely and indicated her willingness to participate. She understood the reason for the special re-evaluation was to plan for her transition to the Junior High School, so she did not appear to have test anxiety. She worked diligently throughout the testing period.

Due to Nicole's blindness the Performance section of the WISC–R was not administered. The Verbal subtests will be used as an estimate of her intellectual abilities. Verbal expressive skills were in the superior range. Nicole's performance indicates an excellent command of the English language, both receptively and expressively. She demonstrated superior verbal concept formation and higher level thinking in social problem-solving. There were no true weaknesses noted among her verbal abilities.

In summary, Nicole's performance on the Verbal subtests of the WISC–R indicate superior range intellectual abilities. There were no true weaknesses noted. Her behavior during testing was socially appropriate and cooperative.

School Psychologist

Psycho-Educational Evaluation

Tests Administered

Woodcock-Johnson Psycho-Educational Battery: Tests of Cognitive Ability

Auditory Memory Cluster	%ile *99*	SS *135*
Memory for Sentences	Grade Range *12.9*	
Numbers Reversed	Grade Range *12.9*	

Slingerland Screening Test Form D (large print; typed for written)

Visual Memory	*88%*
Visual Discrimination	*100%*
Visual Memory to Written	*90% items/80% sequencing*

Auditory Memory to Written	*100% items/80% sequencing*
Auditory Discrimination	*100%*

Woodcock-Johnson Psycho-Educational Battery: Tests of Achievement

Reading	GE *5.4*	AE *10-7*	%ile *21*	SS *88*
Word Identification		Grade Range *6.0–7.0*		
Word Attack		Grade Range *4.5–6.0*		
Passage Comprehension		Grade Range *4.5–6.0*		
Mathematics	GE *8.0*	AE *13.5*	%ile *71*	SS *108*
Calculation		Grade Range *8.0–9.0*		
Applied Problems		Grade Range *6.0–8.0*		
Written Language	GE *12.9*		%ile *91*	SS *120*
Dictation		Grade Range *4.5–6.0*		
Proofing		Grade Range *8.0–11.0*		
Punctuation & Capitalization		Grade Range *11.0*		
Spelling		Grade Range *4.5–5.5*		
Usage		Grade Range *9.0–11.0*		

Classroom Reading Inventory (Silvaroli)

Level	Listening Comprehension
8	*100%*

Illinois State Dept. of Education Secondary Informal Reading Inventory

Level	Listening Comprehension
9	*100%*
10	*90%*
11	*80%*

Test of Written Language: Written Language Quotient *100*

Vocabulary	%ile *50*	SS *100*
Thematic Maturity	%ile *75*	SS *100*
Word Usage	%ile *50*	SS *100*
Style	%ile *50*	SS *100*

Testing Interpretation

Learning Modality. On the *Woodcock-Johnson* Auditory Memory Cluster, Nicole's performance indicated superior range functioning for age, grade, and cognitive expectations. Her excellent memory for sentences indicates accurately remembering 15–18 word sentences. Her performance on the auditory reorganization task (numbers reversed) indicates accurately reversing seven digits.

The *Slingerland* was administered with appropriate modifications such as using large print and allowing responses to be typed rather than hand written. Nicole performed adequately on the visual memory (88%) and visual discrimination tasks (100%). She committed one "b-d" reversal and one letter transposition on the visual memory task. All number and letter sequences were accurate. The auditory discrimination and auditory memory tasks revealed excellent abilities, when paired with a written response the tasks, though adequate, were much more difficult.

Reading and Listening Comprehension. Nicole's performance in reading large print on the *Woodcock-Johnson* was below age, grade, and cognitive expectations (GE 5.4) as compared to non-vision impaired students. Word identification was at grade expectancy (grade range 6.0–7.0), while word attack and passage comprehension were below expectancy (grade range 4.5–6.0). These skills were significantly impacted by Nicole's legal blind visual status. The word attack subtest indicated gaps in knowledge. She tends to substitute short vowel sounds; experienced some difficulties with double vowels, sounds of "y," silent letters. She appeared to understand basic syllabication rules. She read orally fluently through the 4th grade level. At higher levels her performance indicated frustration as she did not use phonics or syllabication as decoding strategies, relying on context clues. This is not unexpected as Nicole's primary mode of learning is auditory with heavy reliance on context clues for meaning.

Nicole was administered Informal Reading Inventories to assess listening comprehension. At the 8th grade level on the *Silvaroli* she scored 100% on the comprehension questions asked. At the 11th grade level on the *Illinois,* she scored 80% experiencing difficulty with questions requiring sequence of events and vocabulary definition. These results indicate that if all other reading skills were commensurate, Nicole could be expected to read silently at the 11th grade level with instructional level comprehension. A significant difference exists between her listening comprehension and her reading performance level, again due to the visual impairment.

Mathematics. On the *Woodcock-Johnson* Mathematics Cluster, Nicole performed above-average range for age and grade expectations (GE 8.0). Her performance indicates that she understands all of the basic mathematical processes; and computation of fractions. On the applied problems, she demonstrated a good understanding of computation of two-step problems. She experienced some difficulty with problems involving time, percentages, and fractions. Nicole appears to have good reasoning ability and very good abstract computation skills.

Written Language. On the *Woodcock-Johnson* Written Language Cluster, Nicole scored in the superior range for age and grade expectations. Proofing, punctuation and capitalization, and word usage were areas of strength. Spelling and dictation appeared to be areas of weakness. Problems in phonics were obvious in the spelling subtest as Nicole attempted to write the words.

The *TOWL* was administered to assess application of knowledge of written language rules. Nicole's overall performance indicated low average functioning for age expectations. On the Style subtest, capitalization and punctuation of skeleton sentences, Nicole's performance was in the average range for age expectations. On the Word Usage subtest, Nicole's performance was in the average range for age expectations experiencing a few problems using irregularly formed plurals, pronoun antecedents, and verb tenses.

The Vocabulary and Thematic Maturity subtest scores were determined by analyzing a spontaneous creative writing sample. On the Vocabulary subtest, Nicole performed in the average range for age expectations. She utilized numerous higher level vocabulary words in her creative story. Nicole's performance on the Thematic Maturity was above age expectations and consistent with cognitive expectations. She wrote an integrated story utilizing the three stimulus pictures. She wrote in paragraphs using correctly capitalized and punctuated sentences. Nicole's story incorporated pictorial relationships, reasons for environmental hostility, original names for characters, and the role of the spacelings. There were many spelling errors.

Summary. Nicole experiences visual processing deficits due to her legal blind status. Her auditory processing skills appear excellent for age, grade, and cognitive expectations; and adequate when a written response is required.

Academically, Nicole experiences expected discrepancies between reading and listening skills. Reading word attack skills and comprehension are weaker than expected for age and grade expectations. Her performance indicates a reliance on context clues rather than using phonics or structural analysis. Nicole displayed superior listening comprehension skills, five years above grade expectations. On the written language assessment, Nicole experienced difficulty in spelling. Usually Nicole uses the Spell-Check on her computer, so in daily work uses higher level vocabulary than this written sample evidenced. Informal assessment of her written language product indicated excellent thematic maturity (story structure), correct use of capitalization and punctuation, and use of paragraphs. Calculation and applied problems are above-average for age and grade expectations.

Educational Diagnostician

Social and Emotional Evaluation (Informal)

Nicole is a delightful sixth grade student who has been legally blind since infancy. She uses large print, computer, and recorded compressed speech as her means of learning. She has always been in the regular classroom with resource or consultative assistance.

Social Perspective-Taking. Nicole appears to have good social perspective-taking skills. At school she readily volunteers to serve as primary grade or special education tutor. She shows much patience and concern for those experiencing academic and/or physical difficulties. She makes inferences about people's characteristics from the way they act and treat others. Though, legally blind she is very perceptive to facial expressions and gestures of those near her, and to the nuances in people's voices. Due to legal blindness, she experiences difficulty interpreting by voice alone interactions involving people at distances. She is developing more insight into the reciprocal nature of social interactions. She, also, has a very realistic view of her handicapping condition and its limitations.

Social Regulation and Moral Development. Nicole is making good progress in this area. She conforms to several sets of rules regarding moral codes and behaviors (e.g., family, church, school, peers). She is aware of the nuances of written and unwritten rules and codes of conduct. Nicole learns through indirect socialization techniques such as discussion. She, however, cannot read (due to legal blindness) cues such as facial expressions and gestures across the room and misses many of the unspoken interactions among people (e.g., teasing, expressions of anger). In getting along with people, Nicole has learned not to jump to hasty conclusions. She regulates her behavior according to social rules and rule-governed play. She experiences difficulty in competitive athletic games (e.g., kickball), however, she enjoys trying and depends on team cheering for cues about when and where to run. She understands that appropriate behavior differs in various social settings. Nicole is very sensitive to negative reactions of others.

Social Problem-Solving. Nicole is very good in solving social problems presented orally. Due to vision limitations, she experiences difficulty in social group situations depending on vision for cues on interpersonal interactions. She understands cause-effect reasoning, and solves social problems.

Social Relationships: Peers. Nicole appears to be a well-adjusted sixth grader. She has a small group of special social friends with whom she spends most of her free time. Through the peer-tutor program, she has become acquainted with students in many grade levels. She does not engage in many unsupervised activities, but does enjoy going to the Mall to walk around with friends on Saturday afternoons. She belongs to a number of clubs such as Girl Scouts and Rainbow Girls and participates actively in their activities.

Self-Competence/Self-Evaluation. Nicole appears to have a good concept of self and accepts her handicapping condition. She displays good self-control and is even tempered. She is very skilled on the computer and this has provided her much status among peers for word processing, graphics, and games. She is a good student and is proud of the work she does. There are few things that she really wants to do that she cannot do in some fashion.

Summary. Nicole demonstrates good social and emotional development. She is making continued progress in social perspective-taking, social regulation, social problem-solving, and social relationships. She appears to be a well-adjusted pre-adolescent girl.

Elementary School Counselor

Adaptive Behavior: Vision Functioning Evaluation (Informal Assessment)

History. Nicole is a sixth grade student who was diagnosed legally blind in infancy. She has received special education services from teachers and coordinators of the Vision Impaired Program since diagnosis. She attended a special preschool for VI children which focused on using residual sight, orientation and mobility, motor skills, and readiness skills. During primary grades enrolled in the regular elementary classroom, Nicole received daily VI Resource Services to help her learn to use the computer, to develop listening comprehension skills and use of recorded compressed speech, to learn basic academics including reading large print books and writing (manuscript and cursive) on special wide line paper. As Nicole became proficient at these skills, the VI Services were reduced. Currently, she receives only periodic itinerant or consultative services.

Daily Activities. Nicole makes good use of her vision. She is totally self-sufficient in self-help and grooming skills. At home she is learning cooking, housekeeping, and care of her clothing. Her parents have taught her many skills using the computer including budgeting and simple accounting.

Travel. Nicole seldom goes anywhere unaccompanied. In the future (Junior High & High School), since she will not be able to drive, she needs to learn to use the Mass Transit System to get around the city to recreation and employment sites. Throughout public school years, she will have special education bus service to and from school. She does occasionally go on an errand for mother to the corner grocery store, but there is no street crossing required. On Saturday afternoons she accompanies her friends around the Mall. Nicole will need some assistance getting to and from classes at the Junior High School. With so many students in a rush and all of the halls looking very similar initial orientation will be difficult.

Recreation. Nicole relies on the computer for much of her recreational activities (e.g., games and graphics). She enjoys recorded books and music. She belongs to several organizations and participates in those activities. For health and well-being, Nicole needs to include frequent swimming or other aerobic-type activity into her daily/weekly routine.

School. Nicole functions very successfully at the elementary school that she has attended since kindergarten, and can easily go from place to place independently. She will need VI services at the Junior High School to learn the new environment. There will, also, need to be consultative VI services to her teachers to help with any needed curriculum modifications. Her class schedule needs to be decided now to order books and specialized materials (e.g., science beakers with large print measuring marks).

Summary. Nicole's adaptive behaviors are good. As she moves to the Junior High School, she will need increased VI Services at least initially to ensure a smooth transition. Consultative VI Services will be provided to her teachers to plan any curricular adaptations. She will need help getting to and from classes until she learns the new environment. This can probably be facilitated by an organized system using peers.

Consultant, Vision Impaired Program

Evaluation Summary

Nicole is a 12 year, 5 month old legally blind sixth grade student, who attends regular classes. She is functioning on grade level using large print books, recorded textbooks, and a computer with an oversized monitor.

Cognitive assessment indicates Nicole is functioning within the superior range intellectually. She demonstrated superior verbal concept formation and higher level thinking in social problem-solving. She displayed an excellent command of the English language both receptively and expressively. She demonstrated excellent auditory processing abilities. Visual skills using large print materials are adequate but much slower than auditory.

Academically, Nicole evidenced significant differences among her listening comprehension skills (11th grade level) and reading skills (GE 5.4). This is expected due to her limited vision and to her superior auditory skills and performance using recorded compressed speech. Phonics and related spelling skills are weak, however, use of context clues was very strong. Mathematics, calculation and applied problems (GE 8.0) are above average for age and grade expectations. She understands and uses all mathematics algorithms in calculation and applied problems. Written expression skills in isolation and in spontaneous creative writing reveal average to superior range functioning with spelling as the only weakness.

Nicole appears to be well adjusted socially and emotionally. She engages in social perspective-taking, social regulation, social problem-solving, and appropriate social relationships. Adaptive behavior appears appropriate to age, grade, and environment. Vision-related problems that Nicole may encounter at the Junior High School include the logistics of changing classes and securing specific materials and supplies. Plans need to include development of skills for independence in traveling, and inclusion of an active recreational activity such as swimming.

Case Manager

DIAGNOSIS: Vision Impaired

Chapter Two

CASES OF COMMUNICATION IMPAIRED STUDENTS

Communication encompasses the areas of speech and language. Speech is concerned with correct articulation, voice, and fluency, in other words, the vocal production or the sounds of communication. Language, however, primarily concerns the content of communication. Language includes the structure of words (phonology, morphology), the structures of sentences (syntax), the meanings of words and sentences (semantics), and the social use of language to communicate (pragmatics). Communication impairments, then, involve a dysfunction in speech and/or language.

Speech and/or language impairments are associated with numerous other handicapping conditions including hearing impairment, mental retardation, and learning disabilities. Thus, a specific intelligence quotient is not specified, but the child's overall developmental functioning is compared to his/her language functioning to determine if a discrepancy exists.

Preschool Age/Grade: See Cara & Diana
Primary Age/Grade: Megan
Intermediate Age/Grade: Jason
Secondary Age/Grade: See Kirk

EVALUATION REPORT
MEGAN

Age: 5 years, 10 months
Grade: Kindergarten
Date: May , 19____

Background and Educational Concerns

Reason for Referral

Megan is a 5 year, 10 month old kindergarten student attending Jackson Elementary School. The kindergarten teacher has been concerned about Megan's expressive language development. Megan seems eager to please, is alert, smiles a lot, and attempts tasks presented. She appears to understand most of the directions given to her, but does very little communicating. At first the teacher assumed Megan was shy as she would not communicate during Show & Tell, Puppet Time, or Language Experience period. During play time, she joins the play of a group of children, participates in the activities, may laugh and enjoy herself, but communicates mostly by gestures. When she does communicate, her soft voice and articulation errors make her difficult to understand. Her teacher has recommended retention in kindergarten for the next academic year.

Health

Immunizations are current. School health records indicate a physical examination prior to kindergarten with no concerns noted.

Vision and Hearing Screenings

School vision and hearing screenings indicate average range acuities.

Speech and Language Screenings

School speech screening indicated normal range voice, articulation, and fluency. Language screening indicated deficits in expressive language.

Socio-Economic and Home Information

English is the language of the home. Megan has two younger sisters, ages 3 years and 1 year. Father is a self-employed plumber, and mother baby sits five other preschoolers. The family lives in their own home, a small brick house with large yard, in a working class neighborhood. The parents seem pleasant and interested in Megan's school progress, but feel that she is just very shy which makes her seem backward. She has always played with the other children in the home. Megan did not attend preschool. There appears to be no social or economic deprivation.

CURRENT MULTIDISCIPLINARY EVALUATION

This evaluation includes the following assessments: cognition, perception, memory, speech/language, academic achievement, and behavior.

Psychological Evaluation

Tests Administered

Wechsler Preschool and Primary Scale of Intelligence (WPPSI)

Verbal IQ	*84*	Performance IQ	*119*	Full Scale IQ	*101*
Information	*6*	Animal House	*14*		
Vocabulary	*6*	Picture Completion	*10*		
Arithmetic	*12*	Mazes	*12*		
Similarities	*6*	Geometric Design	*14*		
Comprehension	*7*	Block Design	*14*		

Developmental Test of Visual-Motor Integration (Beery) CA *5-10* AE *6-1*

Testing Interpretation

Megan is a small, friendly 5 year, 10 month old kindergarten student. She entered the testing situation somewhat shy, holding her head down and swinging her body side-to-side not making eye contact. Rapport was readily established and she smiled and nodded that she was ready to try the activities.

Results of the *WPPSI* indicate a significant difference among verbal expressive and psychomotor skills invalidating the full scale score as representative of Megan's abilities. Megan's overall verbal performance was at the upper limits of the borderline range of intelligence, while psychomotor performance was in the superior range of intelligence. Verbal expressive skills weaknesses include making statements of learned facts, practical knowledge and social judgment, verbal concept formation, describing relationships between facts and ideas, defining vocabulary. She performed within the average range on tasks requiring manipulation of numbers. Megan's psychomotor skills revealed primarily high average to superior range functioning in visual-motor planning, visual analysis and reproduction of abstract designs, and nonverbal judgment. On the *Beery,* Megan functioned above age expectations on visual-motor integration tasks.

In summary, Megan demonstrates cognitive functioning potential at the superior level as indicated by her superior psychomotor skills. Her test performance indicates significant weakness in verbal expressive skills at the upper limits of the borderline range. A language evaluation is recommended.

School Psychologist

Language Evaluation

Tests Administered

Peabody Picture Vocabulary Test-Revised (PPVT-R) CA *5-10* IQ *101*
Language Screening Sample CA *5-10* AE *4.6-5.0*

Testing Interpretation

Receptive Language. Megan's performance on the *PPVT-R* indicated average range functioning in receptive language. An informal test of receptive language indicated that she knows right from left, number concepts to 10, follows a 3-step command, can repeat four digits, provides definitions of familiar objects, and can remember a sentence of 10 words in length. She experienced difficulty with some relational concepts including words of quantity (e.g., most, least; medium sized; widest). Receptive language functioning appears to be at the 5–6 year level.

Expressive Language. On an informal expressive language sample, Megan's performance indicated functioning in the 4-6 to 5-0 age range. Emerging skills included possessives (my, mine, his, her), pronouns (I, me, it), simple past tense, and conjunctions (because). Acquired skills included simple adjectives (comparative, superlative), prepositions (on, in, with, of, for, to, at, up), uncontracted coupla (am, is, are, was, were), articles (a, the), and conjunctions (and). Megan's mean sentence length was 4.5 words. She asks and understands questions beginning with "who, what, when." She can point at pictures and tell a simple story, but needs great encouragement. Her expressive language functioning is approximately 14 months delayed for age.

In summary, receptive language appears to be within normal limits. Expressive language appears to be deficit in excess of one year.

Speech/Language Pathologist

Psycho-Educational Evaluation

Tests Administered

Woodcock-Johnson Psycho-Educational Battery: Tests of Cognition

Visual Perceptual Speed	GE *1.4*	AE *6-7*	%ile *86*	SS *116*
Auditory Memory Cluster	GE *1.0*	AE *5-10*	%ile *50*	SS *100*

Woodcock-Johnson Psycho-Educational Battery: Tests of Achievement

Preschool Skills Cluster	GE *1.0*	AE *6-0*	%ile *52*	SS *101*

Slingerland Screening Test: Prereading, Revised

Near Point Copying	*adequate*
Far Point Copying	*adequate*
Visual Memory-Choice Response	*80%*
Visual Discrimination	*90%*
Visual Memory to Written	*90%*
Auditory Memory to Written (Letters)	*88%*
Auditory Discrimination	*75%*
Auditory Visual Association-Pictured Object	*100%*
Auditory Visual Association-Comprehension	*75%*
Auditory Visual Association-Letter Knowledge	*88%*
Auditory Visual Association-Sound Symbol	*90%*

Chart of Normal Development (Informal Assessment)

Gross Motor Skills (5–6 year level)
- Runs forward, backward & on toes.
- Walks forward, backward, up & down stairs, on balance beam.
- Hops, skips, gallops, jumps.

Fine Motor Skills (5–6 year level)
- Cuts out simple shapes.
- Draws triangles, squares, circles.
- Prints numerals 1–5.
- Colors within lines.

- Catches, tosses & bounces ball.

Weaknesses: None

Play Skills (5–6 year level)

- Plays games with rules.
- Builds with blocks; plays with clay.
- Likes table games.
- Rides bike.

Weaknesses: 4 to 5 year level

- Dramatizes Stories.
- Plays with puppets.

Cognitive Skills (5 to 6 year level)

- Counts objects in a set 1–20.
- Sorts by color, size, shape.
- Matches capital & lower case letters.

- Writes 1st name.

Weaknesses: None

Social Skills (5–6 year level)

- Takes responsibility.
- Respects authority.
- Engages in cooperative play.
- Shows concern and sympathy.

Weaknesses: 4 to 5 year level

- Engages in role play (no language)
- Chooses own friends.

Cognitive Skills (4–5 year level)

- Retells story from picture book.
- Uses time concepts—yesterday.
- Makes simple predictions.
- Asks many "why" questions.
- Shows cause-effect understanding.
- Tells nature of object (describes it).
- Names objects, tells use.

Testing Interpretation

Learning Modality. Megan's performance on the *Woodcock-Johnson* visual perceptual speed tasks indicated above-average functioning for age and grade expectations, but commensurate with psychomotor abilities. On the visual matching task (visual discrimination of numerals), Megan accurately discriminated one digit, two digit, and three digit numerals. On the spatial relations task she scored above-average attempting many more items than expected, but with an accuracy of 73%.

Megan's performance on the *Slingerland* indicated adequate near-point and far-point copying. She reversed a letter and experienced some difficulties with letter formation and copying a diamond, in general, she was able to accurately copy the designs, numbers, and letters. Megan's visual processing skills of visual memory-choice response (letters), visual discrimination, and visual memory with a written response are all strong skill areas.

Though not as strong as visual skills, auditory skills appear to be adequate. Megan's performance on the *Slingerland* auditory memory to written task revealed only one error, a "b-d" reversal. On the auditory discrimination task Megan experienced difficulty with medial short vowels. On the auditory memory tasks, Megan listened to directions or a paragraph and pointed to a picture or letter as her response. This task did not require her to respond orally and her performance was adequate to excellent. On the *Woodcock-Johnson* auditory memory tasks, Megan scored within the average range for age expectations accurately remembering and repeating seven word sentences and reorganizing (numbers reversed) 2 digit sequences.

Developmental Skills. On the *Woodcock-Johnson* Preschool Skills, Megan's performance indicated average performance for grade expectancy. She correctly identified all of the letters presented, but did not read any of the words. She responded age-appropriately to applied mathematics problems with understanding. Megan understands one-to-one correspondence, used the picture clues to assist in calculation, and appears to understand the concepts of addition and subtraction. Though not a part of the subtest, she correctly answered two of the calculation problems indicating a concept of number symbol association and abstract computation with sums to three. On dictation, she accurately wrote the letters requested in either upper or lower case form.

The informal developmental skills assessment indicated that Megan was functioning within age expectancy in developmental areas that do not require expressive language. However, in developmental areas that require verbal expressive skills, Megan experiences significant deficit functioning within the 4–5 year level or lower. Social deficits include interactions and role play with peers that require verbal exchanges. While she is eager to make friends, these interactions depend on some verbal communication. Cognitive deficits that are a result of deficits in expressive language include retelling stories, making predictions, asking questions, describing objects and telling their functions. Play skill development is deficit in expressive language areas.

In summary, Megan does not appear to have any significant visual or auditory processing deficits. She appears to possess age-appropriate prereading skills, academic, and developmental skills unless the skill involves verbal expressive responses and interactions. Megan appears significantly deficit in verbal expressive language.

Educational Diagnostician

Classroom Behavioral Observations

In the classroom, Megan is alert and friendly. She smiles and interacts with other children sharing toys and engaging in similar activities. In social situations, she responds so expressively facially that it is difficult to determine that she is not interacting verbally. However, during intensive expressive language activities, Megan tries to be invisible. Her facial animation is gone. She appears very shy and withdrawn. She brings an item for Show & Tell, but only wants to show. During puppet time, she will interact in one or two word responses. When asked to retell a story, she becomes so embarrassed and upset that she is unable to do the task. Her only behavioral concerns involve expressive language and verbal interactions.

Resource Room Teacher

Evaluation Summary

Megan is a 5 year, 10 month old kindergarten student. Her cognitive potential appears to be at the superior level as indicated by psychomotor skills. Verbal expressive skills are a significant weakness at the upper limits of the borderline range. Visual motor integration skills are a strength.

Language evaluation indicated age-appropriate receptive language, and severely deficit expressive language. Her expressive language appears to be in excess of one year deficit for age and grade expectations, but several years deficit for cognitive expectations. Academically, Megan possesses adequate visual and auditory processing, and prereading and academic skills. She possesses age appropriate developmental skills except in areas involving expressive language. Cognitive skills, social skills, and play skills are all negatively impacted by deficit expressive language skills.

Behaviorally, Megan is age-appropriate. She is facially expressive, so the lack of language use is not immediately noticeable. She is motivated and attempts all school activities, but has a very difficult time with any activities involving expressive language.

Case Manager

DIAGNOSIS: Language Impaired (Expressive)

Chapter Three

CASES OF HEARING IMPAIRED STUDENTS

"Both deaf and hard-of-hearing persons are hearing impaired". (Jones, 1992, 63) The hard-of-hearing person has a significant hearing loss, but through special adaptation uses hearing to develop speech and language skills (Heward & Orlansky, 1988). The hearing impairment of a deaf person is so severe that s/he is not able to use hearing to understand speech and language.

Preschool Age/Grade: Cara
Primary Age/Grade: See Jeff
Intermediate Age/Grade: Jason
Secondary Age/Grade: Kirk
See also: Sam

EVALUATION REPORT
CARA

Age: 1 year, 6 months
Grade: Infant
Date: December , 19____

Background and Educational Concerns

Reason for Referral

Cara is a 1 year, 6 months old child referred to the Child Find Clinic for evaluation and consideration for services in the Two-Year-Old Program for Handicapped Children. She has previously received services from a program for visually impaired infants.

Health

Parents report Cara's health is good. Medical records have been requested to outline background information. Currently, Cara is taking no medication. She has had immunizations appropriate to her age level.

Visual History

Records have been requested from the family ophthalmologist and from Children's Hospital regarding the status of the Visual Evoked Response testing completed shortly after birth. Cara has a congenital visual impairment.

Auditory History

Records have been requested from Children's Hospital regarding results of the Brainstem Evoked Response Audiometry, information regarding the behavioral testing, and specific information regarding the hearing aids.

Socio-Economic and Home Information

English is the language of the home. Father is an engineer with an airplane manufacturing company. Mother, educated as an elementary school teacher, cares full-time for Cara and her new baby brother, who is nonhandicapped. The family lives in a renovated century-old home in an exclusive neighborhood. Parents are adjusting well to Cara's handicapping conditions. There is no economic deprivation.

CURRENT MULTIDISCIPLINARY EVALUATION

This evaluation includes the following assessments: cognition, vision, hearing, communication, motor, and social development.

Psychological Evaluation

Test Administered

The Callier-Azusa Scale (Cognition) CA *18 months* MA *16–18 months*

Testing Interpretation

Cara is an infant brought to the Child Find Clinic for evaluation. Parents report that she is blind and hearing impaired. She wears hearing aids. Cara was observed by the diagnostic team as she played with toys. Parents provided additional information.

Cara anticipates routine events from environmental cues (e.g., putting on snowsuit means go in the car, putting on bib means time to eat). She realizes that an object continues to exist after she drops it and will "look" for it. She is able to differentiate between sizes of objects by feeling. Cara will push other toys out of the way searching for the one object she wants. She crawls or scoots around in search of an object out of reach. She is in constant motion exploring the environment.

Cara vocalizes similar sounds in response to familiar words, and attempts to approximate words. She localizes the source of sound by turning her head directly toward the source. She will manipulate a musical toy until it makes noise, then lay her face against the toy to hear it better. She imitates familiar gestures such as banging two items together (e.g., blocks, cups). She can imitate a new sequence of behaviors when each behavior in the sequence is part of her repertoire. She also attempted to imitate complex gestures composed of familiar schemas (e.g., she shook the soft rattle, then banged it on the tambourine).

Cara shows much curiosity about objects. She has devised an exploratory system composed of three steps: (1) She shakes the object and puts it to her ear to listen, (2) She puts the object into her mouth to taste and feel, and (3) Almost simultaneously, she is feeling the object with her hands. All of these exploratory behaviors are performed in such a rapid systematic fashion that it takes observing numerous times before the observer is certain what she is doing.

Cara has mastered some very sophisticated combinations of skills. She has discovered that if she puts her face into a plastic bowl and yells that she can hear the echo. She demonstrated good fine motor control by opening a band-aid box and reaching in to get a cracker. She has learned to tactilely use many body parts including her head in searching for items. Emerging skills include learning the sign to represent "eat," and to understand the correspondence between the parts of a three-dimensional representation (doll) and parts of her body.

In summary, Cara appears to be functioning cognitively at the 16–18 months level or within the average range of cognition. Cara understands object concept, imitation, anticipation, object permanence, causality, object constancy, and intentional behavior appropriate to her developmental level. However, in view of her sensory handicaps, blindness and hearing impairment, this evaluation is considered to minimally represent her skills and abilities. Her actual cognitive potential may be closer to the superior or gifted ranges.

School Psychologist

Vision Evaluation

Tests Administered

Informal Optometric Assessment

Testing Interpretation

Cara was brought to the Child Find Clinic by her parents for evaluation. Electrodiagnostic testing at age 3 months revealed "markedly abnormal VER (Visual Evoked Response) consistent with very poor vision."

At this screening, Cara did not demonstrate a protective blink reflex to an object moved quickly toward her eyes, nor to a bright light presented. OKN was not elicited. The pupils reacted very sluggishly to direct light stimulation. Cara did not spontaneously fixate a penlight, flashlight, transilluminated light or toys or other visual stimuli. She did seem to slightly "alert to" and move her eyes "in the direction of" a moving pinwheel (reflective) illuminated by a flashlight.

No eye contact, no spontaneous fixation, no tracking were observed, however, Cara seemed to manifest light perception and possible light projection. The electrodiagnostic findings and the results of this screening indicate legal blindness status at this time. Vision records have been requested from Children's Hospital and the family ophthalmologist.

Optometrist

Hearing Evaluation

Tests Administered

Impedance Test
Behavioral Audiometry

Testing Interpretation

Cara was seen for a hearing evaluation as part of her Child Find Clinic assessment. Requests have been sent to Children's Hospital for copies of her Brainstem Evoked Response Audiometry testing.

Cara's hearing was assessed by observing behavioral responses to various auditory stimuli presented in a sound field. The testing was administered while Cara was wearing her hearing aids. Results were as follows:

Stimulus	*Hearing Level*	*Response*
Monitored Live Voice	25dB	Localization
Squeaky Toy	25dB	Smile
Raggedy Ann Rattle	25dB	Localization
Happy Apple	25dB	Reached toward sound
Cricket Noisemaker	25dB	Cessation
Bicycle Horn	30dB	Startle

Impedance test for middle ear function shows normal tympanograms for both ears. Hearing appears adequate for the reception of speech and language. Cara appears to get good benefits from her hearing aids.

Educational Audiologist

Communication Evaluation (Informal)

Receptively, Cara appears to be functioning at approximately the 7–9 months developmental level. Cara localizes sound by turning her head toward the source of the sound. She can manipulate a musical toy until it makes noise. Mother indicates that Cara has discovered that if she puts her face into a plastic bowl and yells that she can hear the echo. Cara understands the signs "eat" and "drink." If she is holding two items, one in each hand and you say "bang bang," she will clap them together.

Expressively, Cara appears to be functioning at the 7–9 months developmental level. Cara vocalizes similar sounds in response to familiar words, and attempts to approximate words. She says "mama" and "dada" as specific names. She frequently talks to herself, babbling and making various noises. She is learning the signs for "eat," and "drink."

Speech/Language Pathologist

Motor Evaluation

Tests Administered

Brigance Diagnostic Inventory of Early Development
Informal Development Assessment

Testing Interpretation

Gross Motor Skills. Cara appears to be functioning at the 10–14 months level in gross motor skills. She walks around furniture holding on. For brief periods, she will stand alone unaided. She pulls to stand using furniture, and she pulls from sitting to standing by rotating her trunk segmentally. She walks toward an adult when holding on to both hands. Cara sits alone with her arms free to play, scoots forward on her bottom, and pivots on bottom while sitting. She enjoys four-point crawling, and rocking back and forth while in the crawling stance. Cara is very tiny and quite agile.

Fine Motor Skills. Cara appears to be functioning within the 13–18 months range in fine motor skills. She can open a band-aid box and remove a cracker using pincer grasp. Mother keeps a small band-aid box with crackers in her purse for Cara. She opens and closes simple containers, places objects in containers and dumps them out. Cara bangs two objects together. She uses a rattle to bang on a tambourine. She holds objects in one hand while trying to pick up others. She uses arms and hands to hold larger objects.

Self-Help Skills: Eating. Cara feeds herself finger foods. She chews appropriately. She lifts a cup by the handle, but needs help getting it to her mouth for a drink. She grasps a spoon and tries to bring it to her mouth. She appears to be functioning at the 12–18 months level in eating skills.

Self-Help Skills: Dressing. Cara assists in dressing by holding out her arm for the sleeve. She takes off her shoes and socks, and plays trying to put her shoes back on. Cara is functioning at the 12–18 months level in dressing.

Self-Help Skills: Toileting. Cara is being time trained. She does not like wet or soiled clothes and will fuss to be changed. She sits on the potty and plays with musical toys. Cara is functioning at the 12–18 months level.

Tactile Development. Cara's tactile development appears to be at the 36 month level. She explores objects with fingers, and plays with soft-textured materials such as pudding. She responds to tactile stimulation of her arm or leg by moving the stimulated limb. Cara recognizes familiar objects by touching and handling. When she is tired or feels stressful she seeks her pacifier and blanket. She differentiates among objects tactilely, putting objects in her mouth to feel, and feeling with fingers. She prefers her Happy Apple toy and will pick up toys, feel them, and put them down, hunting until she finds it. Cara is very curious, constantly exploring.

Physical Therapist

Social Development

Test Administered

The Callier-Azusa Scale (Social Development)

Testing Interpretation

Interaction with Adults. Cara appears to be functioning within the 18–24 months range in interactions with adults. She responds to person-to-person contact, studies adults tactilely, responds to adults' voices, and initiates interactions with adults. Cara loves to be swung back and forth, and indicates that she wants to continue the activity. Cara differentiates familiar and unfamiliar adults by voice and tactile exploration. She is able to initiate interactions vocally when she wants an adult to help (e.g., change her diaper, find a toy). She stops briefly when told "no."

Peer Interaction. Peer interactions appear to be at the 6 month level. Cara responds to peers and touches them to explore. However, since she is so tiny most children play too rough. Mother indicated that Cara is not often around other children. She does show much interest in her baby brother. She localizes when he cries, stops to listen, then crawls toward the sound.

Interactions with the Environment. Cara appears to be functioning at the 9–12 months level in interactions with the environment. She exhibits rudimentary control of her behavior by vocalizing to exhibit discomfort, fatigue, hunger. She appears to have rudimentary differentiation of her behavior, for example, she exhibits different vocalizations, and rhythmically rocks back and forth. She appears to possess rudimentary differentiation of the environment by expressing preferences for particular foods. She reacts to frustrating situations by yelling and kicking her foot. She responds to noticeable changes in her environment by exploring. Cara shows evidence of possessing finer differentiations of her environment when she anticipates a familiar event, and seeks her pacifier and blanket when she is tired or upset.

Educational Diagnostician

Evaluation Summary

Cara is a one year, six month old child evaluated at the Child Find Clinic. Current psychological evaluation indicates that Cara is functioning cognitively at the 16–18 months developmental level or within the average range for age expectations. She has some understanding of object concept, imitation, anticipation, object permanence, causality, object constancy, and intentional behavior. It is felt that this is a minimal estimate of Cara's cognitive potential because she is blind and hearing impaired. Cognitive potential may be closer to superior or gifted ranges.

Cara's developmental skill levels are as follows:

Developmental Skills	*Functioning Level*
Cognition	16–18 months
Receptive/Expressive Language	7–9 months
Gross Motor	10–14 months

Fine Motor	13–18 months
Self-Help (Feeding, Dressing, Toileting)	12–18 months
Tactile	36 months
Social Skills	
Adults	18–24 months
Peers	6 months
Environment	9–12 months

Cara is an amazing child who performs at or above age expectations in many areas. Blindness and hearing impairment interfere with her overall development most notably in the areas of language (9 months deficit), gross motor skills (4–8 months deficit), social interactions with peers (1 year deficit), and exploring the environment independently (6–8 months deficit).

Visually, Cara appears to be legally blind. At this screening, there was no eye contact, no spontaneous fixation, and no tracking. Cara seemed to manifest light perception and possible light projection. Cara wears hearing aids and appears to get good benefits from them. With hearing aids her hearing appears adequate for the reception of speech and language. Middle ear function appears normal.

Case Manager

DIAGNOSIS: Deaf-Blind and Language Impaired

EVALUATION REPORT
JASON

Age: 11 years, 0 months
Grade: 4th grade (retained in kindergarten)
Date: April , 19___

Background and Educational Concerns

Reason for Referral

Jason is an 11 year old student attending Monroe Elementary School. He is functioning academically in the lower third of his class. He failed reading and health the third quarter, and received I's in social studies, science, and language. His other grades were M's. Jason seems to have difficulty remembering and following a sequence of directions. He needs a great deal of repetition. Jason has difficulty grasping new concepts. Some of his difficulty seems to be his lack of confidence and low frustration tolerance.

School interventions have included remedial instructions (2 years reading and 1 year math). He is involved in group and individual counseling at school. The school has initiated this evaluation because of Jason's failure to make adequate progress in major academic subjects.

Health

Immunizations are current. Jason has a history of otitis media and upper respiratory infections. This past winter he missed several weeks of school due to severe otitis media and sinus infection.

Vision Screening

Jason has mild myopia for which glasses have been prescribed. He does not like to wear his glasses and needs to be reminded to use them.

Hearing Screening

Jason failed the hearing screening test. Referral was made to the school district audiologist.

Speech and Language Screenings

Jason receives speech and language therapy twice a week.

Behavior History

Most of Jason's behavior problems seem related to his academic frustration. He does not start a task without saying that he doesn't understand it or he can't do it. He becomes very frustrated over small things. Jason constantly wants teacher one-to-one help. He often does things to get attention. He usually follows the rules as long as nothing upsets him. Jason usually turns his work in on time, but disregards the quality or accuracy. He does not work well with others. Children who sit by him often ask to be moved. Jason blames others for his actions and views others as not liking him and being unfair. The group therapy session which Jason attends deals with frustration and stress management.

Socio-Economic and Home Information

English is the language of the home. Jason lives with his parents and an older brother in a working class neighborhood. His father is a mail carrier and his mother is a beautician in a neighborhood shop. There does not appear to be economic deprivation.

At home Jason behaves best for his father. He can follow directions, but often needs repetition and explanation. He constantly seeks attention. When faced with frustration, he will ask his father for assistance. Jason needs lots of praise and encouragement. Jason seems to be easily distracted.

There is some competition between Jason and his older brother, but this seems to be within normal limits. He enjoys sports and often plays group sports in the neighborhood. He has one special friend. Jason does seem to have difficulty making and keeping friends, and he will admit occasionally that others do not like him. The parents seem pretty understanding of their sons and try to provide the support they need and yet teach them independence and responsibility. Both Jason and his brother have daily and weekly chores around the house and yard.

CURRENT MULTIDISCIPLINARY EVALUATION

This evaluation includes assessments in hearing, intelligence, perception and memory, speech and language, academic achievement, behavior, and social and emotional development.

Hearing Evaluation

Tests Administered

Impedance Testing
Behavioral Audiometry

Testing Interpretation

Impedance tests for middle ear function indicated normal (both ears) tympanograms, thus, currently Jason does not have otitis media. Behavioral audiometry indicated a mild to moderate hearing loss with the following results:

Unaided Ear	5% Warble Tones						
	125	250	500	1K	2K	4K	8K
Left	35	35	35	40	45	50	45
Right	35	40	40	40	45	45	45

Loaner hearing aids were used on a trial basis. A hearing aid evaluation indicated functioning within the 20–30 dB HL. Recommend repeated monitoring to determine which hearing aids produce the greatest benefits. Results indicate that Jason would receive good benefits from hearing aids.

Educational Audiologist

Psychological Evaluation

Tests Administered

Wechsler Intelligence Scale for Children-Revised (WISC-R)

Verbal IQ	*79*	Performance IQ	*99*	Full Scale IQ	*88*
Information	*7*	Picture Completion	*10*		
Similarities	*6*	Picture Arrangement	*11*		
Arithmetic	*7*	Block Design	*10*		
Vocabulary	*6*	Object Assembly	*11*		
Comprehension	*7*	Coding	*7*		
Digit Span	*5*				

Bender Gestalt Test CA *11-0* AE *7-6 to 7-11* Limit Testing *8-6 to 8-11*
Detroit Test of Learning Aptitude Oral Directions AE *6-3*

Peabody Picture Vocabulary Test-Revised (Form L) (PPVT-R)
CA *11-0* AE *9-0* Stanine *3* SS *84*

Testing Interpretation

Jason, an eleven year old, fourth grade student, displayed some unusual behaviors during the testing sessions. He seemed to be in an agitated state of anxiety related to test taking which may have interfered with optimal performance. He picked at his fingernails, which were already badly bitten. He periodically shook his head in a strange way and made noises with his mouth as he worked. He seemed unaware of doing these things.

Jason was overly concerned about whether each of his responses were correct or not, frequently trying to see what the examiner was writing. He made comments such as "I'm trying, I really am". "You think I can get this right?" "Is this past my age?" "That's wrong, I know that's wrong". He interpreted any change in the examiner's facial expression as an indication that he was doing poorly.

Jason tended to approach tasks in a highly impulsive and disorganized manner. Instead of thinking about a problem and planning a solution, he would jump right in with an impulsive trial and error approach, quickly becoming frustrated and wanting to give up. The examiner's attempts to reduce anxiety by giving support, encouragement, and reassurance were only minimally successful.

Jason was administered the testing while wearing his loaner hearing aids. Results of the *WISC-R* indicated a significant difference between borderline verbal expressive skills and average range psychomotor skills. Jason is considered to be within the average range of intellectual functioning. No significant differences were noted among his verbal expressive skills. Weaknesses were noted in verbal concept formation and ability to recognize and describe essential relations between objects or ideas, and in defining words. He also experienced difficulty with tasks requiring auditory memory and auditory sequencing. The entire area of verbal expressive language abilities is weak.

Overall, psychomotor skills were within the average range of intellectual functioning. Relative strengths were noted in nonverbal judgment using picture cues, visual-motor perception and coordination, and part-whole relationships in assembly tasks. Relative weakness was noted in ability to learn symbols and shapes and to recreate them quickly.

On the *Detroit,* auditory sequencing of verbal directions, Jason scored almost 5 years deficit for age expectations. He had great difficulty attending to, remembering, and executing the multi-step directions.

On the *Bender,* Jason scored significantly below age expectations. Limit testing resulted in only a minor improvement. Rotation, distortion, and integration errors were noted. Jason's performance was characterized by heavy pencil pressure, spontaneously abandoned designs, and disorganized placement. These features are often characteristic of a youngster who is disorganized and is experiencing difficulty controlling his impulses.

Jason's performance on the *PPVT-R,* a test of receptive language, was significantly below age expectations at the 9 year level. The receptive language score is commensurate with *WISC-R* verbal test scores.

In summary, Jason appears to be a youngster of average intellectual ability. He experienced significant weaknesses in verbal reasoning and auditory sequencing of directions. Visual motor skills are also an area of difficulty. Behavioral difficulties such as poor impulse control, lack of self-confidence, disorganization, and a high level of failure anxiety appear to be interfering with his test performance as well as his classroom functioning.

School Psychologist

Psycho-Educational Evaluation

Tests Administered

Wepman Auditory Discrimination Test	*85%*
Slingerland Screening Test Form C	
Far-Point Copying	*Poor to Fair*
Near-Point Copying	*Fair*
Visual Memory	*89%*
Visual Discrimination	*100%*
Visual Memory to Written	*55% items/82% sequencing*
Auditory Memory to Written	*44% items/44% sequencing* (Form C)
	76% items/67% sequencing (Form B)
Auditory Discrimination	*71%*

Woodcock-Johnson Psychological Battery: Tests of Cognitive Ability

Visual Perceptual Speed	GE *4.3*	AE *9-6*	%ile *47*	SS *99*
Auditory Memory Cluster	GE *3.8*	AE *8-10*	%ile *14*	SS *84*

Woodcock-Johnson Psychological Battery: Tests of Achievement

Reading Cluster	GE *3.1*	AE *8-2*	%ile *5*	SS *75*
Word Identification	Grade Range 3.0–4.0			
Word Attack	Grade Range 2.0–3.0			
Antonyms-Synonyms	Grade Range 3.0–4.0			
Analogies	Grade Range 2.0–3.0			
Passage Comprehension	Grade Range 2.0–3.0			
Math Cluster	GE *3.4*	AE *8-7*	%ile *14*	SS *84*
Quantitative Concepts	Grade Range 3.0–4.0			
Calculation	Grade Range 3.0–4.0			
Applied Problems	Grade Range 2.5–3.5			

Durrell Analysis of Reading Difficulty (Listening Comprehension)

Level	*Comprehension*
1st grade	*86%*
2nd grade	*75%*
3rd grade	*70%*
4th grade	*65%*

Test of Written Language (TOWL): Written Language Quotient *70*

Vocabulary	%ile *2*	SS *69*
Thematic Maturity	%ile *3*	SS *72*
Word Usage	%ile *9*	SS *80*
Style	%ile *5*	SS *75*

Test of Written Spelling (TWS)

Predictable Words	*Unpredictable Words*	*Total*
GE *2.8*	GE *3.1*	GE *3.0*
SA *8-5*	SA *8-5*	SA *8-5*
SQ *75*	SQ *75*	SQ *75*

Testing Interpretation

Learning Modality. Jason's performance on the *Woodcock-Johnson* visual matching of numbers and spatial relationships indicated average functioning for grade expectations. On the *Slingerland* (3rd–4th grade level), Jason experienced difficulty with near- and far-point copying. However, visual memory (89%) and visual discrimination (100%) were areas of strength. The item analysis on visual memory with a written response revealed a significant number of spelling errors, but the sequence of items was adequate. The visual modality is Jason's strongest learning channel, but he experiences difficulty with written responses and handwriting.

The auditory channel, when aided, is considerably weaker than the visual channel. On the *Slingerland* (3rd–4th grade level), Jason scored minimally adequate on auditory discrimination (71%), and severe deficit on the auditory memory with a written response task on items and sequencing. When administered the *Slingerland* (2nd–3rd grade level), Jason's score was still in the deficit range. Auditory memory of sentences and numbers on the *Woodcock-Johnson* was below age and grade expectations.

Reading and Listening Comprehension. Jason's overall performance in reading indicated severe deficit for age and grade expectations. Relative strength was noted in word identification, and antonyms and synonyms (3.0–4.0 grade range). Severe weaknesses in word attack (2.0–3.0 grade range) indicate that Jason probably learned to read by a sight-word method. Deficiencies in word attack are also noted in phonology and morphology. Oral reading was characterized by "word-by-word" reading. Jason did not use his limited word attack skills or context clues in decoding unknown words. Passage comprehension measured with a cloze test and analogies (2.0–3.0 grade range) were areas of significant weakness. Reading is an area of significant weakness for age, grade, and cognitive expectations.

Listening comprehension instructional level was minimally at the 3rd grade level. Jason was able to answer fact and literal level questions, but experienced difficulty with vocabulary and inference questions.

Written Expression. Jason, a left-handed writer, experienced significant difficulty in the area of handwriting (e.g., near- and far-point copying, spontaneous writing). At times he wrote with so little pencil pressure as to render his writing so light it was barely readable. Jason was able to write better when given a pen with a rubber gripper. His pencil grasp was inappropriate, and accommodation of handedness to paper was poor causing inappropriate slant. Difficulties with handwriting and lack of automaticity negatively impacted all tasks requiring coordinating thought and a written response.

Jason's spelling performance on the *TWS* indicated severe deficit functioning for age, grade, and cognitive functioning. His performance on predictable words (phonetic) revealed difficulties in short vowel substitutions, letter transpositions, and final syllables. His performance on unpredictable words (nonphonetic) was similar to that on predictable words. Jason's spelling is commensurate with his word attack performance.

Jason's overall performance in written expression on the *TOWL* indicated functioning in the severe deficit range for age, grade, and cognitive expectations. His performance on the Word Usage subtest, commensurate with verbal cognitive functioning, indicated deficits in past tense verbs and pronoun antecedents. His performance on the Style subtest (capitalization and punctuation) was in the severe deficit range with difficulties in capitalizing proper nouns and in using apostrophes and commas.

In the expressive writing sample, Jason's use of higher level vocabulary words was in the severe deficit range for age, grade, and cognitive expectations. He utilized only three higher level vocabulary words in his story. His performance on the Thematic Maturity subtest was in the deficit range for cognitive expectations, the story was too short and the level was extrapolated. His story utilized four of the twenty items evaluated.

Informal assessment of the written language sample indicated that Jason did not write in complete sentences. Generally, he wrote in complete thoughts, which were not punctuated. He attempted to use his very limited knowledge of capitalization and punctuation, but the result was limited in accuracy. His sample reflected difficulties using verb tenses, noted in the Word Usage subtest.

Mathematics. Jason's performance in mathematics indicated deficit functioning for age, grade, and cognitive expectations. His primary area of weakness appeared to be in the area of applied problems (2.5–3.5 grade range). Knowledge of quantitative concepts and calculation appeared evenly developed in the 3rd to 4th grade range. Jason appears to understand the algorithms of addition and subtraction, though he made several errors due to lack of attention to signs. He appears not to understand the algorithms of multiplication, division, and computation of fractions. Calculation errors indicate basic fact deficits.

On the applied problems subtest, Jason experienced difficulty with abstract calculation. He appeared to need visual input to help solve problems. Abstract calculation resulted in computation errors, though questioning revealed correct process. He appears to understand relationship concepts that indicate which mathematical process to utilize. He appears to understand the process required to calculate two-step problems, thought he did not compute any accurately. He experienced extreme difficulty in sorting through extraneous information to locate the facts needed for problem solving, and with calculating money, time, and measurement problems.

Educational Diagnostician

Speech and Language Evaluation (Informal Therapy Assessment)

Speech

Jason has received speech therapy since 1st grade. Currently, his therapy focuses on the correct articulation of /s/, /z/, /s-blends/, /kt/, /tr/. His articulation is at least 90% intelligible.

Language

Jason has received language therapy since 1st grade. His expressive language is characterized by difficulties in structure (phonology, morphology, syntax), semantics, and pragmatics.

Structure. Jason's expressive language is characterized by adequate simple structure, adequate sequencing, and appropriate responses. Phonology and morphology deficits are obvious in his poor functioning in spelling (predictable-phonetic) at 2.8 GE on the *TWS* and in the reading word attack functioning at 2.0–3.0 grade range on the *Woodcock-Johnson.* Jason's difficulty with word usage especially passives, negatives, questions, pronoun antecedents, and complex or unusual wording of sentences is also indicated on the *TOWL.* Jason understands simple and negative imperative, and active declarative (regular noun) sentences. He experiences difficulty with some interrogatives, inherent negation, and sentences using the "if-then" and "neither-nor" sentence patterns.

Semantics. Jason experiences difficulty in semantics as evidenced on the *WISC-R* where he revealed significant weaknesses in verbal reasoning and higher level verbal comparison and contrasting. Auditory comprehension of oral directions on the *Detroit* indicated functioning 5 years deficit for age expectations. The *PPVT-R* indicated receptive language at 2 years deficit for age expectations. Additionally, listening comprehension at 2nd grade level indicated difficulty with higher level questions including inference, cause-effect, and evaluation. Additionally, Jason experiences difficulty with figurative language (e.g., idioms, puns, metaphors), words with multiple meanings, and sarcasm. This difficulty with vocabulary also affects all content subjects with specialized vocabularies including mathematics.

Pragmatics. The area of pragmatics is very difficult for Jason. He understands and uses the conversational skills of initiating, maintaining, and concluding conversations. He continues to experience difficulty in social conversations, blaming others and engaging in negative verbal interactions with peers. He is concerned that others don't like him. He is improving in therapy in his ability to read body language and understand that his negative body language interferes with friendship-making.

Speech and Language Therapist

Behavior Evaluation

Test Administered

Quay Timed Observations: (1) Science: On-Task 73%
(2) Independent Language Work: On-Task 53%
(3) Social Studies: On-Task 80%
(4) Independent Morning Work: On-Task 93%

Testing Interpretation

Jason's behavior was observed on four separate days using the Quay observation method. During a science period Jason was on task 22 of 30 segments or 73% of the time. Off-task behaviors included verbalizing to his neighbor, disturbing others, playing with his pencil and making noises. Twitching was noted 6 out of 30 segments.

The second observation was during an independent language work period. Jason was observed on-task 16 of 30 segments or 53% of the time. Off-task behaviors included vocalizations, turning around in seat, getting out of seat, and looking at observer. During this observation, Jason appeared very frustrated. He argued with the teacher when asked to erase his paper, however, he was getting up to get the eraser at the same time that he verbally argued about it. Jason appeared to have difficulty sitting still in his seat at all times during this observation and continually sought peer and adult approval.

The third observation was during social studies period, when Jason was on-task 24 out of 30 segments or 80% of the time. Off-task behaviors included tapping a pencil on his knee, making faces at students, vocalization, and turning around in his seat.

The fourth observation was during independent morning work and Jason was on task 28 of 30 segments or 92% of the time. Off-task behaviors included tapping a pencil and turning around in his seat.

Informal observations in the classroom and hallways indicate that Jason is active and consistently verbalizes to teachers and peers. Often in the classroom he appears to be very frustrated and lacks self-confidence. He often verbalizes, "I can't do it" or "I don't understand." On the playground, Jason is somewhat more aggressive than the other children; however, he is able to follow directions adequately from those who are supervising. In Physical Education, he is able to follow the teacher's directions.

The classroom teacher reports that work is turned in on time, but sometimes only partially finished. In science he is able to complete all short term assignments, but is inconsistent if more than three days are given to complete the work. Task completion in social studies is inconsistent. He either completes all or none of the assigned work.

Resource Room Teacher

Social and Emotional Development (Informal Counseling Assessment)

Jason's social development appears delayed. He experiences difficulty with social perspective-taking continuing to view everything from his own point-of-view. He does not show concern for the feelings of others, and cannot make social inferences about how his behavior will affect others.

Jason does not learn through indirect socialization techniques such as discussion and sitting next to a student who exhibits the behavior the teacher desires. Jason experiences difficulty understanding that appropriate behavior differs in various social settings. Social problem-solving is an area of difficulty for Jason. He is not sensitive to social problems and social consequences. He does not understand cause-effect relationships in social situations.

Social interactions with peers are difficult for Jason. Since he lashes out and blames classmates, they are not anxious to try to make friends with him. Jason's actions and words suggest a negative academic self-concept. He appears outer-directed and does not accept responsibility for his social or academic difficulties. He appears to fear failure, but his behaviors in the classroom often result in failure.

Currently, small group and individual counseling focuses on stress reduction, appropriate ways of dealing with stress and frustration, and appropriate interpersonal skills.

Guidance Counselor

Evaluation Summary

Jason is an 11 year old 4th grade student who was retained in kindergarten. His overall cognitive functioning is within the average range of intelligence with borderline verbal expressive skills and average psychomotor skills. Visual processing appears to be a weakness with a written response. Auditory memory with an oral or written response appears significantly deficit.

Hearing evaluation indicates that Jason experiences a mild to moderate hearing loss, but when fitted with hearing aids he functions within the normal range. All testing was administered with hearing aids.

Speech and language assessment indicate functioning at the 6–7 year level. Jason experiences difficulty in structure (phonology, morphology, syntax), semantics, and pragmatics. He experiences difficulty with higher level verbal reasoning and auditory sequencing of directions.

Academically, Jason's functioning in all academics are depressed for both age and grade level, and cognitive expectations. However, in reading, math, and written expression Jason appears to be functioning commensurate with his borderline cognitive abilities. Listening comprehension appears to be a significant weakness, as does, use of written expression mechanics.

Social and emotional behaviors are below expectancy. Jason responds impulsively to both adults and peers and at times appears unaware of his actions. He is often aggressive towards peers in instructional settings. Jason has a difficult time staying on-task and engages in many self-distracting behaviors. He appears to lack organization, motivation, and task focus to complete most assignments especially long term assignments. Jason is often frustrated in the classroom and fears failure, resulting in much anxiety. He lacks social perspective-taking and social problem-solving abilities.

Case Manager

DIAGNOSIS: Hearing Impaired (mild-moderate) and Speech/Language Impaired

RE-EVALUATION REPORT
KIRK

Age: 17 years, 1 month
Grade: Ungraded Special School
Date: May , 19____

Background and Educational Concerns

Reason for Referral

Kirk is a 17 year, 1 month old student enrolled in an ungraded special day school for handicapped adolescents. He was diagnosed hearing impaired (moderate) as an infant and has received special education services since diagnosis. Parents have been adamant that he attend the special school for hearing impaired and deaf students. He wishes to be considered for programming that includes 1/2 day academics and 1/2 day vocational training. Kirk's current programming includes regular academics, remedial reading, speech and language therapy, and prevocational areas. He is also receiving programming to assist with social and emotional development focusing on stress management, self-control, and appropriate interactions with others. This is a routine re-evaluation.

Health

Immunizations are current. School health physical last fall indicated no specific concerns. Hearing impairment is a result of meningitis as an infant.

Vision Screening: Normal visual acuities.

Hearing

Kirk experiences a moderate sensorineural hearing impairment. He receives good benefit from his hearing aids.

Speech and Language

Kirk has received speech and language therapy since infancy. He is language delayed in all areas.

Behavioral History

Though not severely behavior disordered, Kirk does experience some difficulties in interpersonal relationships. He frequently misreads body language including facial expressions, gets angry, and has a temper tantrum before the situation can be explained. He has a very low frustration tolerance and a "chip on his shoulder."

CURRENT MULTIDISCIPLINARY EVALUATION

This evaluation includes assessments in intelligence, hearing, speech, language, social communication, academic achievement, and vocational skills.

Psychological Evaluation

Test Administered

Wechsler Adult Intelligence Scale-Revised (WAIS–R)

Verbal IQ	*78*	Performance IQ	*105*	Full Scale IQ	*92*
Information	*6*	Picture Completion	*10*		
Vocabulary	*5*	Picture Arrangement	*9*		
Arithmetic	*7*	Block Design	*12*		
Similarities	*5*	Object Assembly	*12*		
Comprehension	*5*	Coding	*11*		
Digit Span	*5*				

Testing Interpretation

Kirk is a 17 year, 1 month old hearing impaired adolescent who attends a special day school (adolescent wing) for academic and vocational training. He entered the testing situation somewhat reluctant. He had experienced reevaluation previously so understood the process. He was cooperative and worked diligently throughout the testing.

Results of the *WAIS–R* indicate overall average range intellectual functioning with borderline verbal expressive skills and average range psychomotor skills. There were no significant strengths or weaknesses noted among verbal expressive skills. Relative strength was shown in ability to manipulate number concepts. Kirk functions primarily at the concrete level, higher level thinking and abstract concepts are difficult for him.

Average range psychomotor skills revealed no significant strengths or weaknesses. Relative strength was noted in visual-motor perception and coordination, and simple assembly skills. He performed adequately in the ability to learn shapes and symbols and to recreate them, and in nonverbal judgment using picture cues.

In summary, Kirk is a hearing impaired (moderate) adolescent functioning within the average intellectual range with borderline verbal expressive skills and average range psychomotor abilities.

School Psychologist

Hearing Evaluation

Tests Administered

Impedance Testing
Electroacoustic Analysis of Hearing Aids
Behavioral Audiometry

Testing Interpretation

Kirk was diagnosed in infancy as having a moderate sensorineural hearing loss in both ears as a result of bacterial meningitis. Upon diagnosis he was fitted with hearing aids and has received good benefit from them. Kirk communicates primarily using speech, however, he also signs to communicate with his mother and deaf friends.

This is Kirk's annual hearing evaluation. His previous 10 evaluations have all indicated consistent results. Impedance testing for middle ear function revealed normal tympanograms. An electroacoustic analysis of hearing aids indicated they were functioning properly. A hearing aid evaluation in the sound field indicated functioning at 25dB HL. Kirk receives good benefit from his hearing aids.

Educational Audiologist

Communication Evaluation

Tests Administered

Speech and Language Assessment (Informal)
Social Communication for Handicapped Adolescents (pre/post tests)

Testing Interpretation

Speech. Kirk experiences difficulty with articulation, fluency, and intonation. He experiences some difficulty articulating the more difficult consonants /t/, /v/, /l/, /s/ and the more difficult blends using those consonants. His articulation is approximately 85% intelligible to strangers. Current therapy has also focused on understanding and interpreting, and using intonation to assist in conveying messages.

Language. Kirk functions primarily on the concrete level in verbal expression and understanding. All areas of language including phonology, morphology, syntax, semantics, and pragmatics are areas of difficulty for Kirk. Severely deficit functioning in reading and written expression substantiate this weakness. Word identification and word attack at the 2.0–3.0 grade range on the *Woodcock-Johnson* indicate deficits in phonology and morphology.

Word usage is an area of significant deficit. Kirk is functioning at approximately the 6–7 year level having mastered personal pronouns, verbs (present, future), prepositions, adverbs, and possessives. He experiences difficulty with pronoun antecedents, conjunctions, past tense verbs, complex or unusual wording (e.g., Is it not so . . .). Kirk has mastered many sentence types, but experiences difficulty with sentences with past tense verbs, wh-questions, negatives, and if-then conjunctions. He experiences difficulty with figurative language (e.g., idioms), analogies, synonyms, homophones.

Social Communication. Kirk has received small group intervention using *Social Communication Skills for Handicapped Adolescents.* He understands and spontaneously uses conversational skills involving listening strategies, speaker and listener rules, conversational rules; and initiating, maintaining, and concluding a conversation. He continues to experience some difficulty recognizing and understanding emotions and the appropriate expression of emotions. He has shown considerable improvement in reading and using body language to communicate, and in understanding and using vocal inflection. Kirk has shown improvement in interpersonal skills, but continues to experience difficulty in appropriate ways to handle teasing, sarcasm, complaints, criticism, and false accusations. The whole area of interpersonal relationships and conflict management continue to be problematic for Kirk.

Speech/Language Pathologist

Psycho-Educational Evaluation

Tests Administered

Woodcock-Johnson Psycho-Educational Battery: Tests of Cognitive Ability

Visual Perceptual Speed Cluster	GE *6.4*	AE *11-8*	%ile *16*	SS *85*
Visual Matching of Numbers (100%)		Grade Range *5.0–6.0*		
Spatial Relations (89% items, 78% puzzles)		Grade Range *8.0–10.0*		
Auditory Memory Cluster	GE *2.3*	AE *7-7*	%ile *<1*	SS *<65*
Memory for Sentences		Grade Range 2.0–3.0		
Numbers Reversed		Grade Range 1.0–2.0		

Slingerland Screening Test Form D

Far-Point Copying	*Good*
Near-Point Copying	*Good*
Visual Memory	*100%*
Visual Discrimination	*100%*
Visual Memory/Written Response	*75% items/91% sequencing*
Auditory Discrimination	*71%*
Auditory Memory/Written Response	*67% items/75% sequencing*

Woodcock-Johnson Psycho-Educational Battery: Tests of Achievement

Reading	GE *2.5*	AE *7-8*	%ile *2*	SS *69*
Word Identification		Grade Range *2.0–3.0*		
Word Attack		Grade Range *2.0–2.5*		
Passage Comprehension		Grade Range *2.0–3.0*		
Mathematics	GE *9.2*	AE *14-8*	%ile *38*	SS *95*
Quantitative Concepts		Grade Range *7.0–9.0*		
Calculation		Grade Range *10.0–11.0*		
Applied Problems		Grade Range *9.0–10.0*		

Wide Range Achievement Test-Revised (Spelling) GE *2.5* %ile *2* SS *69*

Test of Written Language Written Language Quotient *77*

Vocabulary	%ile *16*	SS *85*
Thematic Maturity	%ile *16*	SS *85*
Word Usage	%ile *5*	SS *75*
Style	%ile *1*	SS *65*

Classroom Reading Inventory (Silvaroli)

Listening Comprehension	3rd grade	*70%*
	4th grade	*60%*
	5th grade	*60%*
	6th grade	*40%*

Testing Interpretation

Learning Modality. Kirk's performance on the *Slingerland* (5th–6th grade level) indicated adequate visual discrimination, visual memory, and visual memory with a written response. Near-point and far-point copying were good. On the *Woodcock-Johnson* Visual Matching of Numbers subtest, Kirk correctly responded to all tasks attempted, functioning within the 5.0–6.0 grade range. On the Spatial Relations subtest at the 8.0–10.0 grade range, he correctly answered 89% of the items attempted and 78% of the puzzles, apparently sacrificing accuracy for speed. Essentially the visual learning modality appears to be a good modality for learning.

On the *Slingerland,* auditory discrimination (71%) and auditory memory with a written response (67% items/75% sequencing) indicate barely minimal functioning at the 5th–6th grade level. The items score is negatively impacted by spelling errors. Performance on the Auditory Memory for Sentences (grade range 2.0–3.0) and Numbers Reversed (grade range 1.0–2.0) subtests on the *Woodcock-Johnson* indicate significant deficits for age, grade, and cognitive expectations. The auditory channel is a significantly weaker modality for learning due to his hearing impairment.

Reading and Listening Comprehension. Kirk's performance in reading (GE 2.5) indicates an area of severe deficit for age, grade, and cognitive expectations. Word recognition, word attack, and passage comprehension appear to be evenly developed. Kirk appears to have learned to read by a sight word method as he possesses few phonetic skills and did not attempt to use phonics as a means of decoding unfamiliar words while reading orally. During oral reading, he committed vowel and consonant substitution errors, and did not use context clues effectively in decoding words. He read word-by-word.

Listening comprehension on the *Silvaroli* indicated 3rd grade instructional level. Kirk experienced difficulty with questions dealing with inferences, cause-effect, and evaluation.

Written Expression. Kirk's performance in spelling on the *WRAT-R* (GE 2.5) indicates severe deficiency for cognitive expectations. His primary errors involved vowel substitution. He appears to rely on his visual memory skills in spelling. This performance is commensurate with his performance in other language arts areas.

Kirk's overall performance in written expression on the *TOWL* indicated severe deficit functioning for age and cognitive expectations. Performance on the Word Usage subtest indicates severe deficit functioning in the areas of verb tenses, irregularly formed plurals, and pronoun antecedents. He appears to understand comparatives.

Kirk performed within the severe deficit range on the Style subtest (capitalization and punctuation). He understands basic punctuation (period or question mark) at the end of a sentence and capitalization of proper nouns. He experienced difficulty with punctuation involving the use of commas; periods after initials and titles; and the apostrophe, colon, and hyphen.

On the written language sample, Kirk's performance indicated low average functioning for age and grade expectations. In the story, he utilized ten higher level vocabulary words. His performance on the Thematic Maturity subtest (story content and structure) indicated low average functioning for age and cognitive expectations. Informal assessment of the written language sample indicated that Kirk utilized his basic knowledge of punctuation and capitalization, wrote in complete simple sentences, and attempted to write in paragraphs. He wrote an integrated story with beginning, middle, and ending.

Mathematics. Kirk's overall performance in mathematics indicated average range functioning for cognitive expectations in quantitative concepts, calculation, and applied problems. Kirk appears to understand the algorithms of addition, subtraction, multiplication, and division. He appeared to know the basic math facts. He adds and subtracts fractions requiring a common denominator, and reduced answers. He experienced difficulty with division of fractions.

On the applied problems subtest Kirk's performance revealed good abstract calculation and abstract reasoning ability. He demonstrated an understanding of two-step problems. Kirk experienced some difficulty sorting through extraneous information in word problems to locate facts critical to solve the problem. He demonstrated good ability to calculate problems dealing with money, time, and measurement. He revealed an understanding of the relationship concepts that indicate which mathematical process is required in problem-solving. Kirk experienced difficulty with problems dealing with map skills, percentages, and geometry.

Summary. The visual channel is a strong means for learning. The auditory channel due to hearing impairment is a significantly weaker modality for learning. Academic areas dealing with language (e.g., reading, listening comprehension, written expression) are areas of severe deficit, while mathematics is an area of considerable strength.

Educational Diagnostician

Vocational Evaluation

Tests Administered

Informal Leisure Inventory	*Satisfactory*
Work Behaviors Simulations (Informal)	*Satisfactory*
Daily Living Skills Simulations (Informal)	*Satisfactory*
Informal Social Skills Survey	*Deficits*
Competitive Employment Survival Skills	*95%*
Survival Vocabulary (Informal)	*90%*
Parent Questionnaire	

Reading-Free Vocational Interest Inventory-Revised

Horticulture	%ile *95*	Stanine *8*
Animal Care	%ile *95*	Stanine *8*

Testing Interpretation

Daily Living Skills. Kirk's ability and academic achievement testing indicate that he has the mathematics skills (GE 9.2) to learn to compute family finances, create a budget, balance a checkbook, and compute cost of items in shopping. However, his language arts skills at the 2nd to 3rd grade level indicate that reading and spontaneous creative writing are areas of difficulty. An informal list of survival vocabulary was administered due to his poor reading skills. Kirk appears to know 90% of the survival words and phrases, information signs, safety signs, employment signs, transportation signs, community signs, medical words, and grocery store words.

Parents indicate that at home, Kirk has demonstrated caring for his personal needs independently. He frequently cooks the family meal using numerous appliances, range, and/or microwave oven. Kirk is regularly assigned various housekeeping tasks including vacuuming and dusting, laundry and ironing. His preferred chore is yardwork which involves driving the riding lawn mower.

Many leisure activities are planned around the Deaf Community Center activities including teen dances, roller skating, and ice skating. Kirk seems to prefer solitary rather than team sports.

Personal-Social Skills. Though Kirk does appear to have a fairly good self-concept, he experiences difficulty in interpersonal relationships. He has trouble interpreting people's intentions, controlling his frustration and temper. Social communication has improved due to systematic instruction, but conflict management remains a problem.

Occupational Skills. On the *Vocational Interest Inventory,* Kirk indicated horticulture and animal care as the career areas in which he was most interested. During work behaviors simulations, he demonstrated knowledge of yardwork involving planting and mulching flowers, and yard maintenance (e.g., mowing, raking, disposing of clippings). During summers, Kirk has operated a small business doing yardwork for neighbors. He expressed an interest in working for a plant nursery or landscaping company.

The Competitive Employment Survival Skills (Informal) indicated adequate skills for the public work place. He appears to possess necessary skills to participate in the ½ day academics and ½ day vocational training program. His success will depend on self-control during frustration and appropriate social interactions.

Vocational Teacher

Evaluation Summary

Kirk is a 17 year, 1 month old student attending a special day school for handicapped adolescents. Results of his cognitive evaluation indicate average range intellectual potential with borderline verbal expressive skills and average range psychomotor skills.

Kirk has a moderate sensorineural hearing loss. He gets good benefit from his hearing aids functioning at 25dB HL. He communicates primarily using speech, but he signs to communicate with mother and deaf friends. He experiences deficits in speech articulation, fluency, and intonation. Kirk functions on a very concrete level linguistically and is delayed in all language areas. Social communication is a concern with difficulties in appropriately dealing with teasing, sarcasm, criticism, and conflict management.

Testing indicates the visual channel is a strong learning modality. The hearing impairment significantly reduces his auditory functioning. Academic areas dealing with language arts areas including reading, written expression, and listening comprehension are significantly weak at the 2nd to 3rd grade level. He knows 90% of the survival vocabulary. Mathematics, calculation and applied problems (GE 9.2), are areas of significant strength.

Vocational evaluation indicates the only concern is interpersonal relationships and controlling frustration. Kirk indicated an interest in a career in horticulture or animal care, both of which are outdoors and solitary activities. Work behaviors and daily living skills indicate satisfactory progress. Currently, Kirk possesses the skills to begin the vocational training program.

Case Manager

DIAGNOSIS: Hearing Impaired (moderate) and Speech/Language Impaired

Chapter Four

CASES OF MENTALLY RETARDED STUDENTS

"Most students classified as mildly mentally retarded obtain IQ scores between 50–55 and 70–75; thus, they progress intellectually at one-half to three-fourths the rate of average nonhandicapped children" (Jones, 1992, 82). Individuals with moderate retardation are those who display significant adaptive deficits and are functioning intellectually within 30–35 to 50–55 IQ range (Grossman, 1973). Severely/profoundly mentally retarded students function 3–4 standard deviations below the mean, IQs 30 or less in both adaptive behavior and intellectual functioning (Wolery & Haring, 1989).

MILDLY MENTALLY RETARDED
- Preschool Age: Jaime
- Primary Age: Debbie
- Intermediate Age: Rodney
- Secondary Age: Dallas

MODERATELY MENTALLY RETARDED
- Primary Age: Mark
- Intermediate Age: Vicky
- Secondary Age: Sam

SEVERE/PROFOUND MENTAL RETARDATION
- Primary Age: Jeff
- Intermediate Age: Heather
- Secondary Age: Randy

EVALUATION REPORT
JAIME

Age: 5 years, 5 months
Grade: Kindergarten
Date: February , 19____

Background and Educational Concerns

Reason for Referral

Jaime is a 5 year, 5 month old kindergarten student who was referred for testing by her kindergarten teacher. Jaime is very immature and is unable to do any of the class work expected of kindergarten students. She has a very short attention span and no independence skills. She has very little concept regarding the purpose of school. The teacher aide has worked one-to-one with Jaime since the beginning of school to keep her disruptions of the class to a minimum.

Health

School health records indicate immunizations are current. A physical examination required prior to school entry revealed no specific concerns.

Vision and Hearing Screenings: Normal Range Acuities

Speech and Language Screenings

Informal screening indicates functioning in the 3–4 year range. Voice, fluency, and oral peripheral mechanism are within normal limits. Jaime has acquired articulating single phonemes /k/, /b/, /g/, /r/ and consonant blends /gr/, /mp/, /br/. She speaks in simple active declarative sentences of 4–8 words. She follows 2 step commands and answers who and what questions. She is willing to talk freely to strangers.

Developmental Skills Screening

The *Denver Developmental Screening Test* was administered by the classroom teacher to estimate Jaime's functioning level. Her overall performance indicated functioning within the 3–4 year range. In personal social skills, Jaime dresses with supervision, removes clothing, buttons most buttons, washes and dries face and hands, and feeds herself. Fine motor adaptive skills indicate that she can copy an "0," build a tower of 8 cubes, pick up raisins with pincer grasp, select the longer line. Her gross motor skills are as follows: kicks a ball forward, throws ball overhead, balances on one foot for 2 seconds, jumps, pedals tricycle, hops, catches a bounced ball.

Socio-Economic and Home Information

English is the language of the home. Jaime is the oldest of three children. Her parents own and operate a small jewelry store where they, also, make jewelry of semiprecious stones. The family lives in a townhouse complex of many families with children. The complex has a playground and several swimming pools. The complex, also, has a Latch Key Alternative Recreation Program where parents leave school-age children before and after school with supervision. There appears to be no economic deprivation.

CURRENT MULTIDISCIPLINARY EVALUATION

This evaluation includes the following assessments: cognition, speech and language, motor, self-help, preacademic, and social skills.

Psychological Evaluation

Test Administered

Wechsler Preschool and Primary Scale of Intelligence (WPPSI)

Verbal IQ	*70*	Performance IQ	*65*	Full Scale IQ	*68*
Information	*4*	Animal House	*5*		
Vocabulary	*4*	Picture Completion	*4*		
Arithmetic	*4*	Mazes	*3*		
Similarities	*5*	Geometric Design	*3*		
Comprehension	*3*	Block Design	*4*		

Testing Interpretation

Jaime is a 5 year, 5 month old kindergarten student who appears rather small and immature for her age. She was brought reluctantly to the testing situation by her kindergarten teacher who brought a bag of M & M's for reinforcement. Teacher indicated that Jaime was stubborn and would not work unless rewarded. The examiner regretted this situation because testing behavior could not be observed more naturally and Jaime was encouraged to manipulate the situation.

Results of the *WPPSI* indicated cognitive functioning within the mild retardation range in verbal expressive and psychomotor abilities. No significant differences were noted among the verbal or performance tests. Relative weakness in verbal expressive skills was noted in social judgment. Relative weakness in psychomotor skills was noted in visual-motor planning and following a visual pattern, and geometric designs.

As was expected Jaime refused to work without her reward, but worked quite diligently for primary reinforcement. She experienced difficulty with paper and pencil tasks, and became quite upset that she could not copy designs and follow mazes.

In summary, Jaime is functioning within the mild retardation range of intelligence with little variability among verbal expressive and psychomotor skills. She demonstrated immature and manipulative behaviors.

School Psychologist

Speech and Language Evaluation

Tests Administered

Language Screening Sample (Informal)
Northwestern Syntax Screening Test

Testing Interpretation

On the *NSST,* Jaime's receptive and expressive language appears to be at the 3½ to 4 year level. Jaime can point to pictures of common objects when they are named and identify objects when told their use. She understands questions that begin with "who, what, or where;" and negatives "no, not, can't, don't." Jaime understands size comparatives (big, bigger). Jaime can follow 2–3 stage commands. She is beginning to understand relationships expressed by "if. . . . then or because" sentences.

Expressively, Jaime speaks in simple declarative sentences of 3–5 words. She frequently gives her first and last name, asks what and where questions, and makes negative statements. Jaime uses /s/ on nouns to indicate plurals, uses /ed/ on verbs to indicate past tense, refers to self using the pronouns "I" and "me."

Jaime's voice, fluency, and oral peripheral structures were adequate.

Misarticulations were maturational indicating that Jaime is functioning on the 3–4 year level. She misarticulates /sch/, /ch/, /t/, /sh/, /v/, /l/, /s/, /y/.

Speech/Language Pathologist

Psycho-Educational Evaluation

Tests Administered

Developmental Tasks for Kindergarten Readiness

Subtests	*% Accuracy*
1. Social Interaction	*61%*
2. Name Printing	*0%*
3. Body Concepts: Awareness	*58%*
4. Body Concepts: Use	*80%*
5. Auditory Sequencing	*50%*
6. Auditory Association	*100%*
7. Visual Discrimination	*40%*
8. Visual Memory	*43%*
9. Visual Motor	*13%*
10. Color Naming	*100%*
11. Relational Concepts	*88%*
12. Number Knowledge-Counting	*90%*
13. Number Knowledge-Use	*25%*
14. Number Knowledge-Naming	*70%*
15. Alphabet Knowledge	*35%*

Test of Early Reading (TERA)

Reading Quotient	*66*
Percentile	*5*
Reading Age	*3 years, 3 months*

Testing Interpretation

Testing Behaviors. Jaime is a friendly 5 year, 5 month old kindergarten student. She came to the testing situation reluctantly and displayed significant attentional problems. Jaime's behavior interfered with task focus to the extent that she required primary reinforcers (candy) to continue the testing. She selectively responded to questions and at times refused to comply unless rewarded immediately. Jaime could be refocused with verbal prompts. Once the primary reinforcers were introduced, she refused to work without a reward. However, this evaluation appears to represent her abilities.

Learning Modality. Jaime appears to experience substantial difficulties with both auditory and visual processing. On the auditory association task which requires considerable reasoning, Jaime scored 100% on the kindergarten readiness test. She experienced significant difficulties with auditory sequencing (50%). Visual processing skills are very difficult for Jaime including visual discrimination of letters (40%), and visual memory of letters and designs (43%). Visual-motor skills are a severe deficit (13%).

Jaime used an awkward pencil grasp which appeared to reduce pencil control. She only copied one design, a circle, and it was very poor quality. She could not reproduce any of the other items (e.g., X, square, triangle, diamond). She copied two letters in manuscript, but could not copy the third letter. She tried to write the three numbers, but all were inverted or rotated.

Preacademics. Jaime's academic performance is severely deficit for age and grade expectations. She knows all of her colors by recognition and by name. Jaime rote counted to nine and recognized seven numerals. She has not acquired the concept of one-to-one correspondence (number use 25%). She recognized and named nine alphabet letters (35%). She experienced difficulty naming body parts (58%), but could discuss the use of the body part when named (80%). Jaime could not print any of the letters of her name. She has a good understanding of some basic relational concepts, such as "front-back, up-down" (88%).

Jaime's social interaction score is severely deficit because of a lack of knowledge of her birthday and address, and for her refusal to attempt questions without reinforcement.

Jaime's performance on the *TERA* is in the severe deficit range for age and grade expectations. Her overall reading score was age equivalent (AE) of 3 years, 3 months. The Meaning subtest was Jaime's strongest performance area at AE 4 years, 11 months. Alphabet knowledge was an area of severe deficit at AE 3 years, 11 months. On Conventions, Jaime scored AE 2 years, 5 months, recognizing top and bottom of the page, but not which word she should read first.

Summary. Visual processing (discrimination and memory) appears to be a significant weakness. Visual-motor skills are so weak that Jaime cannot approximate a circle or letters and numbers. Academically, she is functioning below expectancy for age and grade in name printing, body concepts, number recognition and comprehension, alphabet recognition and identification. Personal data information appears severely deficit. Reading readiness skills are significantly weak. An additional concern is Jaime's lack of independence and her manipulative behavior.

Educational Diagnostician

Motor Evaluation

Test Administered

Developmental Checklists for 3-, 4-, and 5-Year Olds

Testing Interpretation

Gross Motor Skills. Jaime appears to be functioning at the 4–5 year level in gross motor skills. She can catch a ball with both hands against her chest and throw a ball with accuracy. She can walk on a balance beam for six feet. She can hop on both feet several times without assistance. Jaime climbs steps with alternate feet holding onto a hand rail, climbs up the slide and comes down, climbs on the jungle jim, and stands on one foot and balances. She runs freely with little stumbling or falling, and skips haltingly. Jaime can ride a tricycle. She can stack blocks vertically and horizontally and creates structures. Emerging skills include hopping on one foot, walking a straight line, bouncing a ball, skipping rope, and descending stairs alternating feet.

Fine Motor Skills. Jaime appears to be functioning at the 3–4 year level in fine motor skills. She places small pegs in pegboards, cuts with scissors, strings beads with ease, rolls clay, puts together a 6-piece puzzle. Jaime can approximate a circle, but she cannot imitate a cross nor draw a diagonal line from corner to corner in a square, nor draw a square. She cannot print letters or simple words or numerals with a pencil or crayon.

Self-Help Skills: Dressing. Jaime appears to be functioning at the 3–4 year level in dressing. She is learning to button buttons, zip zippers, and tie shoes. She can put on her coat by herself. She dresses and undresses with minor assistance and is learning to buckle a belt.

Self-Help Skills: Eating. Jaime appears to be functioning at the 4 year level in eating skills. She eats well with fork and spoon. She can spread soft butter on bread with a knife, but experiences difficulty cutting with a knife. She pours liquids from a small pitcher and serves herself at the table.

Self-Help Skills: Grooming. Jaime appears to be functioning at the 3–4 year level in grooming skills. She bathes with minimum assistance and brushes teeth. She brushes or combs hair, but needs help with barrettes or pony tails. She is independent in toileting.

Physical Education Teacher and Resource Room Teacher

Social Development

Tests Administered

Chart of Normal Development (Informal Teacher Assessment)

Testing Interpretation

Jaime appears to be functioning at the 3½ to 4 year level in social development. Her behaviors are very inconsistent. She is quite manipulative and will not work without an immediate reward. She has no independent skills. Frequently, Jaime is stubborn and will put her head down, cross her arms, and refuse to budge out of her seat. She experiences difficulty with turn-taking and cooperation. She does not engage in dramatic play, but is quite interested and watches.

Jaime experiences difficulty complying with classroom rules and does not want to replace materials after she uses them. She understands that she has personal property, but does not respect the rights of others. Jaime cannot follow multiple and delayed directions or carry out simple errands. She does not seem to understand classroom routines. Jaime needs constant one-to-one supervision due to her immaturity.

Jaime seems to enjoy being around other children and talks to them. She plays only a short time before wanting the toy her peer has, and tantrums to get it. She does not understand the behaviors expected of her as a student. When Jaime is disciplined (time out chair), she does not understand her misdeeds and feels that the teacher is being mean to her. Jaime does not appear to be behavior disordered, but very immature.

Guidance Counselor

Evaluation Summary

Jaime is a 5 year, 5 month old kindergarten student. Current cognitive evaluation indicates functioning within the mild retardation range of intelligence with little variability among verbal expressive and psychomotor abilities. Concern was noted regarding immaturity and manipulative behaviors.

Academically, Jaime lacks many pre-kindergarten skills. Visual processing especially visual-motor responses are severely deficit rendering her unable to copy or write letters, numerals, or designs. She is functioning below age and grade expectancy in number recognition and comprehension, alphabet recognition and identification, personal data information, naming body parts, reading readiness, and behavior. Developmental functioning appears to be at the following levels:

Developmental Skill	*Functioning Level*
Speech/Language	3½ to 4 years
Gross Motor Skills	4–5 years
Fine Motor Skills	3–4 Years
Self-Help Skills	3–4 Years
Social Development	3½–4 Years

Jaime understands "wh" questions, negatives, size comparisons, and can follow 2–3 step commands. She speaks in simple 3–5 word declarative sentences. Jaime's voice, fluency, and oral peripheral mechanism were adequate. Misarticulations are consistent with cognitive functioning level.

Gross motor skills are a strength for Jaime. Fine motor skills appear to be difficult. She cannot use a pencil or crayon to write numbers, letters, or copy designs. Jaime is functioning at the 3–4 year level in self-help skills.

Socially, Jaime has difficulty following classroom rules and in getting along with peers. She is inconsistent in behaviors, and experiences difficulty with turn-taking and cooperation. She seems to enjoy being around other children, but is very immature.

Case Manager

DIAGNOSIS: Mildly Mentally Retarded

EVALUATION REPORT
DEBBIE

Age: 8 years, 3 months
Grade: 1st grade (retained in kindergarten and 1st grade)
Date: May , 19____

Background and Educational Concerns

Reason for Referral

Debbie is an 8 year, 3 month old 1st grade student at Mason Elementary School. She was retained in kindergarten and enrolled in a transitional kindergarten program. She was retained in 1st grade because she had not mastered 1st grade skills. After the second year in 1st grade, Debbie continues to function at a preschool level. The classroom teacher has requested this evaluation to assist in planning Debbie's academic program for next year.

Health

School immunizations are current. Debbie takes dimetapp or sudafed seasonally for allergies. A physical last summer indicated no specific concerns.

Vision and Hearing Screenings: Normal Range Acuities

Speech and Language Screenings

Speech screening indicated functioning 2–3 years deficit with misarticulations of /l/, /r/, /sh/, /v/, /t/, /s/. Language screening indicated functioning 2–3 years deficit with problems with noun and adverb derivations, irregular plurals, questions, and negatives.

Socio-Economic and Home Information

English is the language of the home. Debbie's father is an Army National Guard technician on OH-58 helicopters and her mother sells cosmetics out of the home. They live in an older settled working class neighborhood several blocks from both sets of grandparents. Debbie has two younger preschool-aged sisters at home. There appears to be no economic deprivation.

CURRENT MULTIDISCIPLINARY EVALUATION

This evaluation includes assessments in the following areas: intelligence, perception and memory, academic achievement, speech and language, self-help skills, and social development.

Psychological Evaluation

Tests Administered

Wechsler Intelligence Scale for Children-Revised (WISC–R)

Verbal IQ	*64*	Performance IQ	*65*	Full Scale IQ	*64*
Information	*6*	Picture Completion	*4*		
Similarities	*4*	Picture Arrangement	*5*		
Arithmetic	*3*	Block Design	*4*		
Vocabulary	*5*	Object Assembly	*7*		
Comprehension	*3*	Coding	*3*		
Digit Span	*3*				

Testing Interpretation

Debbie is an 8 year, 3 month old 1st grade student who was retained in kindergarten and 1st grade. She came eagerly to the testing situation to "play games." Rapport was easily established.

Results of the *WISC–R* indicate overall functioning within the mild retardation range with little variation in verbal expressive and psychomotor skills. No significant strengths or weaknesses were noted. A relative weakness in verbal expressive skills was noted in information gained from experience and education. Relative weaknesses were noted in ability to manipulate number concepts, anticipation and judging consequences of behavioral situations, attention, and auditory memory and sequencing.

Relative strength was noted in psychomotor skills in concentration and simple assembly tasks. Weakness was noted in the ability to learn unfamiliar tasks and speed of visual-motor reaction and association of symbols.

In summary, Debbie's testing behavior was appropriate and she attempted to respond to all "games." Her overall cognitive functioning appears to be within the mild mental retardation range with little variability among verbal expressive and psychomotor abilities.

School Psychologist

Psycho-Educational Evaluation

Tests Administered

Test of Early Reading (TERA):	Total Raw Score	*16*		
	Reading Quotient	*<60*	Percentile	*<1*
	Reading Age	*5-2*		

Slingerland Screening Test: PreReading, Revised

Far Point Copying	*weak*
Near Point Copying	*adequate*
Visual Memory—Choice Response	*63%*
Visual Discrimination	*75%*
Visual Memory/Written Response	*50%*
Auditory Memory/Written Response (Letters)	*25%*
Auditory Discrimination	*70%*
Auditory Visual Association (Pictured Object)	*88%*
Auditory Visual Association (Comprehension)	*63%*
Auditory Visual Association (Letter Knowledge)	*25%*
Auditory Visual Association (Sound Symbol)	*25%*

Brigance Diagnostic Inventory of Early Development

Skills Within (+), Below (–) Age/Grade Expectancy

Color Recognition	+
Visual Discrimination	–
Gross Motor Coordination	–
Identification of Body Parts	–
Directional/Positional Skills	–
Personal Data Response	–
Visual Motor Skills	+
Body Image-Picture	–

Brigance Diagnostic Inventory of Basic Skills: Reading Readiness

Skills Within (+), Below (–) Age/Grade Expectancy

Recites Alphabet (Slurs "l, m, n")	–
Recognizes Upper & Lower Case Letters (Auditory Cue)	–
Recognizes Upper Case Letters by Naming (Visual Cue)	–
Recognizes Lower Case Letters by Naming (Visual Cue)	–
Writes Lower Case Letters From Dictation (Mixed Order)	–

Sight Word Recognition: Stop, Go, Color Words	–
Initial Consonant Sounds	–
Initial Sound Symbol	–
Oral Reading Comprehension, Primer Level	–
Oral Reading Comprehension, 1st Grade Level	–
Writes Alphabet in Order	–
Writes Upper Case Letters From Dictation (Mixed Order)	–

Brigance Diagnostic Inventory of Basic Skills: Math Readiness

Skills Within (+), Below (–) Age/Grade Expectancy

Counting to 39	–
Numeral Recognition to 10	–
Writing Numbers in Sequence to 10	–
Counting Objects to 10	–
Joining Sets	–
Ordinal Concepts (first, last, middle)	+

Testing Interpretation

Learning Modality. Debbie was administered the *Slingerland* level that is ordinarily administered to kindergarten-aged students. Her performance on near-point copying and visual discrimination were in the adequate range. She experienced significant difficulties on the far-point copying, visual memory and visual memory to written subtests, auditory discrimination and auditory memory to written (letters) subtests. On the auditory visual association subtests, Debbie scored within the adequate range on pictured objects. She experienced significant difficulties on the auditory visual comprehension, sound symbol, and letter knowledge subtests. A clear learning modality is not established, however, auditory and visual memory with a written response is very difficult.

Readiness: General Knowledge. Debbie's areas of strength at the readiness level (early 1st grade) include the following: quantitative concepts; sorting by color, shape, and size; naming shapes (circle, square, triangle, diamond); use of objects. Her areas of weakness in General Knowledge included directional and positional concepts, knowledge of body parts, time concepts, knowledge of what to do in certain circumstances, community helpers and services. On the Readiness subtests, Debbie's performance indicated adequate visual discrimination; and matching of shapes, upper and lower case letters, and words. She sang the alphabet slurring the letters together. On the *Basic Skills* test, Debbie's performance was significantly deficit for age expectations. She could read some color words (red), some number words (one, two), and some signs (stop, go).

Written Expression. Debbie experienced significant difficulties on the Manuscript Writing test. She can print her first name, age, and phone number. She attempted to print her upper case letters sequentially, but could not. Some letters were omitted, others reversed, transposed, rotated and inverted. She said that she could not write the lower case letters either sequentially or dictated. Debbie could not write a sentence because she lacks the concept of "sentence." The quality of her manuscript writing is poor, revealing difficulties with slant, size, shape, spacing, and alignment.

Mathematics. Debbie's performance in mathematics is significantly better than her reading performance. She counted by rote to 20, recognized numerals through 5, matched quantity with symbol through 5, understood ordinal concepts (first, last, middle), wrote numerals in sequence through 5, and wrote numerals dictated through 5. Her performance indicated no knowledge of addition or subtraction combinations, a significant deficit for 1st grade. Though Debbie recognizes money, she knows the value of only the penny and dime. She has very few time concepts.

Reading. On the *TERA,* Debbie's performance indicated that her reading level is at the 5 year, 2 month level, a significant deficit by 3+ years for age expectations. She experienced difficulties with meaning, alphabet knowledge, and conventions of written language (e.g., right-left orientation).

Summary. Academically, Debbie appears to be functioning at a prekindergarten level in all areas. She does not recite her alphabet by rote, recognize or write the alphabet. She can count by rote to 20, but recognizes numerals only to 5 and matches quantity with symbol to 5. She has no prereading skills and lacks most math cognitive prerequisites. Debbie is functioning at least three years deficit for age expectations.

Educational Diagnostician

Speech and Language Evaluation

Tests Administered

Language Screening Sample (Informal Test)
Informal Receptive and Expressive Language Checklists
Northwest Syntax Screening Test (NSST)

Testing Interpretation

Receptive Language. Debbie's performance on the *NSST* and informal tests indicate receptive language functioning at the 5½ year level. She knows right from left and number concepts to five, understands words of quantity (e.g., more, less, bigger), follows a three-stage command, repeats four digits and remembers a sentence of 10 words in length. She appears to be functioning over 2½ years deficit for age expectancy.

Expressive Language. Debbie's performance on the *NSST* and informal tests indicate expressive language functioning at the 5½ year level. She asks "when, how, why" questions; can tell a story by pointing to pictures and describing the action in multiword sentences. Debbie's mean sentence length is 5–6 words. She has acquired personal pronouns (I, me, it) and possessive pronouns (my, mine, his, her). She uses present and past tense verbs and prepositions (e.g., after, before, into, down, near, over, under). She is beginning to use conjunctions "if . . . so," and irregularly formed plurals. Debbie experiences difficulty with negative sentences and conjunction sentences (e.g., if-then, neither-nor).

Pragmatics. Debbie is a happy little girl and talks freely much of the time. She understands that communication requires turn-taking; gives and receives information; communicates with family, friends, and strangers. She understands initiating and maintaining a conversation, but not concluding a conversation. Debbie understands basic emotions, body language, and vocal inflection accompanying "happy, sad, angry."

Speech. Informal testing indicates that Debbie is functioning on the 5–6 year level in speech skills. She experiences difficulty articulating /t/, /th/, /v/, /l/, /y/, /z/, /zh/, /s/, /kt/, /tr/, /sp/. She correctly articulates most single consonants and consonant blends. Voice, fluency, and oral peripheral structures are within normal limits.

Summary. Debbie appears to be functioning at the 5½ year level in receptive and expressive language, pragmatics, and speech skills. There is little variability among her speech and language abilities.

Speech/Language Pathologist

Social Development

Tests Administered

Informal Social Skills Development Checklist
Informal Self-Help Skills Checklist
Vineland Social Maturity Scale CA *8 years, 3 months* AE *5 years, 8 months*

Testing Interpretation

Self-Help Skills. Debbie appears to be functioning at the 5–6 year level in self-help skills. She is independent in eating: serves herself at the table, spears food with a fork, spreads soft butter on bread with a knife, and knows not to speak with her mouth full of food. Debbie is independent in dressing: buttons buttons (except back), zips zippers, ties shoes, puts on coat and rainboots. She is independent in toileting. Debbie is independent in grooming: bathes independently, washes hands and face, combs and brushes hair but needs help with washing hair, brushes teeth.

Social/Emotional Behavior. Debbie appears to be functioning at the 5–6 year level in social and emotional development. She wants to do what is expected and respects reasonable authority. She is willing to play with most other children in the class, engages with other children in cooperative play, and shares readily. She enjoys role play in housekeeping, in various adult occupations, and on the playground. Debbie plays simple table games and games with rules. She enjoys singing and playing rhythm band instruments. She produces art projects: cutting, coloring, pasting, painting, molding clay.

Emotionally, Debbie is usually happy and will attempt any task given. She cries when she can not do a task that the teacher expects her to do and feels very unhappy if the teacher is angry. Debbie seldom gets angry or has temper tantrums, and has learned to turn to peers for help in completing tasks that she cannot do. Debbie is liked by most children in the class because she is usually happy and chatty. She respects others' property rights. She participates appropriately in group activities.

Classroom Teacher

Evaluation Summary

Debbie is an 8 year, 3 month old 1st grade student who has been retained in kindergarten and 1st grade. Her overall cognitive functioning appears to be within the mild mental retardation range with both verbal expressive and psychomotor skills within that range.

Academically, Debbie is functioning at a pre-kindergarten level. She cannot recite or write her alphabet, and does not possess pre-reading skills. She counts to 20, writes and recognizes numbers to 5, but she has no knowledge of addition and subtraction.

Speech and language evaluations indicate functioning at the 5½ year level in receptive and expressive language, pragmatics, and speech. She has not mastered all morphological and syntax conventions, and experiences difficulty articulating the harder consonant sounds. Pragmatics skills are good.

Debbie's adaptive behaviors, self-help and social/emotional skills appear to be at the 5–6 year level. She is independent in eating, dressing, grooming, and toileting. Socially, she enjoys peers, cooperates and shares. She enjoys most play activities including singing, dancing, role playing, and art work. She is a happy and pleasant child.

Case Manager

DIAGNOSIS: Mildly Mentally Retarded

RE-EVALUATION REPORT
RODNEY

Age: 11 years, 10 months
Grade: Ungraded Intermediate Mildly Mentally Retarded Program
Date: May , 19___

Background and Educational Concerns

Reason for Referral

Rodney is an 11 year, 10 month old student enrolled in a self-contained classroom (mainstreamed for music, art, PE) for intermediate-aged mildly mentally retarded students. He was initially diagnosed in the second grade (repeated kindergarten and 1st grade), when he was functioning at a kindergarten level. This is a routine three year re-evaluation. Placement decisions to be made include continued placement in the intermediate grade program or moving him to the Junior High School program.

Health

School records indicate that immunizations are current. A physical examination for school indicated no specific medical concerns.

Vision and Hearing Screenings

School screenings indicate normal range visual and auditory acuities.

Speech and Language Screenings

Speech screening indicates voice, fluency, and oral peripheral mechanism are within normal limits. Rodney experiences some misarticulations /y/, /th/, /z/, /s/, /sp/, /tr/, however, his performance appears commensurate with cognitive abilities. Language screening indicates functioning at the 6–7 year level in receptive and expressive language.

Socio-Economic and Home Information

English is the language of the home. Rodney has a younger sister in the third grade. Father is a local TV sportscaster, so the family is very involved in attending regional sports activities. Mother is an exercise teacher at a local fitness center. The family lives in a nice apartment in a complex that caters to families. Rodney and his sister are involved in scouting and after-school recreation programs. There appears to be no economic deprivation.

CURRENT MULTIDISCIPLINARY EVALUATION

This evaluation includes the following assessments: intelligence, perception and memory, academic achievement, language, and social skills.

Psychological Evaluation

Test Administered

Wechsler Intelligence Scale for Children-Revised (WISC–R)

Verbal IQ	*65*	Performance IQ	*63*	Full Scale IQ	*63*
Information	*6*	Picture Completion	*4*		
Similarities	*4*	Picture Arrangement	*5*		
Arithmetic	*3*	Block Design	*4*		
Vocabulary	*5*	Object Assembly	*5*		
Comprehension	*3*	Coding	*3*		
Digit Span	*3*				

Testing Interpretation

Rodney is an 11 year, 10 month old student enrolled in an intermediate grade self-contained classroom for mildly retarded students (mainstreamed for music, art, PE, lunch, library, recess). He came to the testing situation somewhat reluctantly with his teacher who introduced us. She gave him words of encouragement and left. Rapport was readily established and he exerted good effort for the testing.

Results of the *WISC–R* indicate overall cognitive functioning within the mildly retarded range with little variability among verbal expressive and psychomotor abilities. Relative strength in verbal expressive skills was noted in information gained from experience and education. Relative weakness was noted in auditory memory and auditory sequencing, concentration, and arithmetic reasoning, and practical knowledge and social judgment.

Relative strength among psychomotor skills was noted in nonverbal judgment, and visual-motor coordination on simple assembly tasks. Relative weakness was noted in the ability to quickly learn unfamiliar symbols and coordinated with a visual-motor response.

In summary, Rodney appears to be functioning cognitively within the mildly mentally retarded range with little variability among verbal expressive and psychomotor skills.

School Psychologist

Language Evaluation

Tests Administered

Language Screening Sample (Informal) Level: *6–7 years*

Northwest Syntax Screening Test (NSST)
Receptive *6 years, 11 months* Expressive *6 years, 8 months*

Boehm Test of Basic Concepts *85% mastery*

Peabody Picture Vocabulary Test-Revised (PPVT–R) MA *6 years, 7 months*

Testing Interpretation

Expressive and Receptive Language. Overall language testing indicates that Rodney is functioning at the 6–7 year level. He speaks in complete sentences of approximately 7 words in length. He can understand and express his thoughts in basic sentence patterns including simple imperative; simple negative imperative; active declarative using present, past, and future tense verbs. He can understand and asks "Wh" questions.

Receptively, Rodney follows three unrelated commands in proper order and understands sequencing of events when told them. He answers questions related to a short story he has just heard; and verbal absurdity is emerging.

Rodney's performance indicates that he has acquired the use of possessives, comparatives, personal pronouns (present, past, and future verbs), simple and regular plural nouns, conjunctions (e.g., but, after, before, if, so), and prepositions (e.g., after, before, near, into). He answers "what happens if" questions, opposites; and understands yesterday and tomorrow.

Pragmatics. Rodney appears somewhat shy. He can take appropriate turns in conversation, and give and receive information appropriately. He communicates well with family, friends, and strangers. He appears to be functioning on the 6–7 year level. Rodney can determine some intentions of persons by vocal intonation and facial expression.

Speech/Language Pathologist

Psycho-Educational Evaluation

Tests Administered

Woodcock-Johnson Psycho-Educational Battery: Tests of Cognitive Ability

Visual Perceptual Speed	GE *1.2*	%ile *0*	SS *<65*
Visual Matching (100%)		Grade Range *1.0–1.5*	
Spatial Relations (90% items, 74% puzzles)		Grade Range *1.0–1.5*	
Auditory Memory	GE *1.0*	%ile *0*	SS *<65*
Memory for Sentences		Grade Range *1.0*	
Numbers Reversed		Grade Range *1.0*	

Slingerland Screening Test Form B

Far-Point Copying	*Discontinued*
Near-Point Copying	*Discontinued*
Visual Memory	*100%*
Visual Discrimination	*88%*
Visual Memory/Written Response	*22%*
Auditory Memory/Written Response	*18%*
Auditory Discrimination	*10%*

Test of Written Spelling (TWS)

	Total	Predictable	Unpredictable
Spelling Age	*5-5*	*5-5*	*5-7*
Spelling Quotient	*<50*	*<50*	*<50*
Grade Equivalent	*1.1*	*1.2*	*<2.4*

Woodcock-Johnson Psycho-Educational Battery: Tests of Achievement

Reading		GE *1.8*	AE *7-0*	%ile *2*	SS *69*
	Word Identification		Grade Range *1.5–2.0*		
	Word Attack		Grade Range *1.5–2.0*		
	Passage Comprehension		Grade Range *1.5–2.0*		
Mathematics		GE *1.1*	AE *6-2*	%ile *1*	SS *65*
	Calculation		Grade Range *1.5–2.0*		
	Applied Problems		Grade Range *1.0*		
Written Language		GE *1.5*	AE *6-8*	%ile *2*	SS *69*
	Dictation		Grade Range *1.5–2.0*		
	Proofing		Grade Range *1.0–1.5*		

Classroom Reading Inventory (Silvaroli)

Listening Comprehension	2nd grade *70%*
	3rd grade *60%*

Testing Interpretation

Learning Modality. On the *Woodcock-Johnson* Visual Perceptual Speed activities, Rodney performed below expectations for cognitive ability. Upon examination, however, these scores may be more due to lack of speed than accuracy. On the visual matching of numbers (1.0–1.5 grade range), he answered correctly 100% of the items attempted. On the spatial relations activity (1.0 grade range), Rodney correctly responded to 90% of the items attempted and 73% of the total puzzles. Auditory memory appears to be a weakness for cognitive ability (1.0 grade range) as he could only remember 6 word sentences and reverse 2 digits.

On the *Slingerland,* Rodney correctly responded to 100% of the selected visual memory tasks. He experienced some difficulty with visual discrimination (88%), primarily "b-d." However, when a written response to visual memory tasks was required, he experienced significant difficulty. Rodney's auditory discrimination was adequate. Auditory memory with a written response was significantly weak (18%), pairing weak auditory memory with very poor visual-motor and handwriting skills. The near-point and far-point copying tasks were discontinued due to the exorbitant time requirements and visual memory of one letter at a time.

Reading and Listening Comprehension. Rodney's overall reading performance on the *Woodcock-Johnson* at GE 1.8 appears commensurate with cognitive expectations. His performance at 1.5–2.0 grade range on all reading tasks indicates no severe discrepancy among reading abilities. Rodney did not use phonics to decode unknown words. He appears to be learning to read by the whole word method.

Rodney's listening comprehension is minimally at the 2nd grade level. On the *Silvaroli,* he responded correctly to 70% of the questions at the 2nd grade level, and 60% of the questions at the 3rd grade level. He experienced difficulty with inference, evaluation, main idea, and vocabulary questions. He could answer literal level fact questions. Rodney did not respond correctly to any of the questions at the 4th grade level.

Mathematics. Rodney's overall performance in math at GE 1.1 appears commensurate with cognitive expectations. Calculation skills (1.5–2.0 grade range) appear to be significantly better than applied problems

(1.0 grade range). He appears to be learning basic facts sums to ten. He cannot compute regrouping problems.

Rodney's performance on the applied problems appeared inconsistent. However, he inaccurately responded to several problems having picture clues in which the answer seemed obvious. Rodney could not compute problems presenting some picture clues and requiring some abstraction. It was not readily apparent whether Rodney's difficulty was in not understanding the concepts of addition and subtraction or whether he did not understand some of the prepositions used to clue the appropriate mathematical process.

Written Expression. Rodney's overall performance in knowledge of written expression mechanics appears commensurate with cognitive expectations. On the dictation subtest (1.5–2.0 grade range), Rodney correctly spelled one word and related one plural. On the proofing subtest (1.0–1.5 grade range), he did not respond correctly to any of the items. On the *TWS,* Rodney's performance was significantly below cognitive expectations. His functioning level at GE 1.1 was achieved by correctly spelling two words. Rodney's lack of phonics skills negatively impacted spelling performance. He experienced "b-d" reversals even though he wrote in cursive. Rodney was not asked to write a story due to lack of automaticity in handwriting, spelling, and written expression mechanics.

Summary. Rodney is functioning significantly below age and grade expectations in all psycho-educational areas. His functioning in many areas is within cognitive expectations. Rodney's major means of learning appears to be the visual channel. He experiences difficulty with auditory memory, and with both auditory memory and visual memory with a written response.

Academically, Rodney appears to be functioning at the 1.5–2.0 grade range in reading and calculation; and at the 2nd to 3rd grade range in listening comprehension. Handwriting, spelling, written expression, and applied problems appear to be areas of weakness at the 1.0 grade level.

Educational Diagnostician

Social and Emotional Development (Informal Assessment)

Rodney has participated with his class for the past two years, twice weekly for 30 minutes daily in informal personal-social development training activities conducted jointly by the classroom teacher and guidance counselor.

Self-Help Skills. Rodney is independent in self-help areas of eating, dressing, grooming, and toileting. He gets around the school and his neighborhood independently.

Social Perspective-Taking. Rodney is making progress in the area of social perspective-taking. He recognizes and shows concern about how others feel and expresses this concern. Since he is functioning at a very literal cognitive level, he experiences difficulty making inferences about the characteristics of people. He has difficulty understanding how other's personality will affect his own behavior (social inferences). He is developing more insight into the reciprocal nature of social interactions. Rodney can not observe himself and others and engage in social comparison.

Social Regulation and Moral Development. Rodney is functioning on a very literal level and experiences difficulty conforming to several sets of rules regarding moral codes and behaviors. He will modify his behavior when directed to do so. He is not aware of the nuances of written and unwritten rules and codes of conduct. Rodney has very little understanding of the social world and does not learn through indirect socialization techniques. He is developing an increased ability to get along with people, to share, and not always insist on his own way. He can engage in rule-governed play as long as the rules are literal and there aren't too many.

Rodney participates in Special Olympics and after-school recreation programs which involve competition and public comparison. He understands appropriate behavior differs in various social settings, and is sensitive to the negative reactions of others. Rodney feels self-shame when he has engaged in inappropriate behavior and is scolded.

Social Problem-Solving. Due to Rodney's low cognitive functioning ability, independent problem solving in any area is beyond his ability. However, through role-playing he is learning some basic ways to solve social problems. His difficulty with cause-effect relationships negatively impacts problem-solving.

Social Relationships: Peers. Most of Rodney's peers are other students in the self-contained classroom and they get along well. In his mainstreamed classes, other students know about his limitations and interact with him as being "special." Most of his interactions with peers are in formal or informal supervised settings, he has few unsupervised interactions with peers.

Rodney dresses similarly to other students. Grooming has been emphasized in his classroom as well as at home. In the weekly small group meetings for "at risk" students with the guidance counselor, Rodney is learning self-control and means of dealing with group pressure and avoiding trouble. Previously, if an admired peer told Rodney to hit someone or pull up a girl's dress, he would do it and "get-in-trouble" with the teachers. Now he is able to evaluate and determine if he would "get-into-trouble."

Summary. Rodney is immature in terms of behaving as a 6th grade student. He has made significant progress in learning socially appropriate behaviors. He remains vulnerable due to his lack of social problem-solving skills. He functions socially more like a 2nd grade student.

Guidance Counselor

Evaluation Summary

Rodney is an 11 year, 10 month old student enrolled in a classroom for mildly retarded students. Current evaluation indicates cognitive functioning is within the mildly mentally retarded range with little variability among verbal expressive and psychomotor skills.

Language evaluation indicates Rodney is functioning at a 6–7 year level in expressive and receptive language which is commensurate with his verbal intelligence scores on the *WISC-R.* He speaks in complete sentences of seven words in length, and understands and uses basic sentence patterns. He has difficulty with age-appropriate pragmatics.

Academically, Rodney's weaknesses in auditory and visual memory with a written response significantly limit his performance. He appears to be functioning at the 1.5–2.0 grade range in all reading areas and calculation; and at the 2nd–3rd grade level in listening comprehension. Spelling, written expression, and applied problems are areas of significant weakness.

Rodney is independent in self-help skills of grooming, eating, toileting, and dressing. Socially, he is immature in social perspective-taking (e.g., social inferences, social comparisons). Social regulation and moral development are at a very literal level. Rodney experiences difficulty with problem-solving (social) and interacting with nonhandicapped same-aged peers.

Case Manager

DIAGNOSIS: Mildly Mentally Retarded

RE-EVALUATION REPORT
DALLAS

Age: 16 years, 10 months
Grade: Ungraded Program for Mildly Retarded Adolescents
Date: October , 19___

Background and Educational Concerns

Reason for Referral

Dallas is a 16 year, 10 months old student who has received special education services since he was eight years old and diagnosed mildly mentally retarded. He is currently enrolled in a Work-Study Prevocational Program studying academics during the morning and learning work skills in an on-the-job placement in the afternoon. This is a routine 3 year re-evaluation.

Health

Immunizations are current. A sports physical examination in August indicated no specific concerns.

Vision and Hearing Screenings

School vision and hearing screenings indicate normal range visual and auditory acuities.

Speech and Language Screenings

Speech screening indicates adequate voice, fluency, and articulation. Dallas speaks in complete sentences of 7–9 words in length and has a fluent, but concrete use of language.

Socio-Economic and Home Information

English is the language of the home. Dallas is the oldest of four children of a TV repairman and a clothing store clerk. The family lives in an older settled neighborhood where Dallas has always lived. Though father works in a TV repair shop downtown, he fixes TVs in the workshop behind the garage and in his spare time works on old cars in the garage. Dallas and his 14 year old brother have learned electronic and mechanic skills from helping their father. Dallas and his brother alternate the yardwork, trash, and other home chores. The garage and workshop appear to be a local "hangout" for the neighborhood boys and men as there is always a group consulting on or working on a car. Dallas plays sports on various teams throughout the year. There appears to be no economic deprivation.

CURRENT MULTIDISCIPLINARY EVALUATION

This evaluation includes the following assessments: cognition, perception and memory, academic achievement, social development, social communication, and vocational assessment.

Psychological Evaluation

Test Administered

Wechsler Adult Intelligence Scale-Revised (WAIS–R)

Verbal IQ	*64*	Performance IQ	*65*	Full Scale IQ	*65*
Information	*3*	Picture Completion	*4*		
Similarities	*5*	Picture Arrangement	*5*		
Arithmetic	*4*	Block Design	*4*		
Vocabulary	*3*	Object Assembly	*6*		
Comprehension	*5*	Coding	*3*		
Digit Span	*3*				

Testing Interpretation

Dallas is a 16 year, 10 month old student currently attending an ungraded adolescent work-study program for mildly mentally retarded adolescents. He entered the testing situation quietly, but alertly. He attempted all items presented. He was not verbally spontaneous, but remained focused on the task at hand.

Current performance on the *WAIS–R* indicates cognitive functioning within the mildly mentally retarded range with little variation among verbal expressive and psychomotor skills. There are no significant strengths or weaknesses noted among abilities. Overall verbal expressive skills fall within the mild retardation range of cognitive functioning with little variability among the subtests. Relative strength was noted in verbal concept formation and the beginning of abstract thinking, and in social judgment. Relative weaknesses were noted in information gained from experience and education, quality of language used, and auditory memory and sequencing.

Dallas's functioning in psychomotor skills appears to be within the mild mental retardation range with no significant strengths or weaknesses. Relative strengths were noted in social alertness and common sense, speed of visual-motor coordination (e.g., assembling small puzzles), and nonverbal judgment. Weaknesses included analysis and reproduction of abstract designs and ability to recognize essential details.

In summary, Dallas's cognitive functioning appears to be within the mild mental retardation range with little variability among verbal expressive and psychomotor skills.

School Psychologist

Psycho-Educational Evaluation

Tests Administered

Slingerland Screening Test, Form D

Visual Discrimination	*86%*
Visual Memory	*90%*
Visual Memory/Written Response	*67% items, 70% sequencing*
Auditory Discrimination	*92%*
Auditory Memory/Written Response	*56% items, 63% sequencing*

Woodcock-Johnson Psycho-Educational Battery: Tests of Cognitive Ability

Visual Perceptual Speed Cluster	GE *4.1*	AE *9-5*	%ile *3*	SS *72*
Visual Matching (94%)		Grade Range *3.0–5.0*		
Spatial Relations (91% items, 90% puzzles)		Grade Range *4.0–6.0*		
Auditory Memory Cluster	GE *4.4*	AE *9-9*	%ile *4*	SS *74*
Memory for Sentences		Grade Range *4.0–5.0*		
Numbers Reversed		Grade Range *3.0–4.0*		

Woodcock-Johnson Psycho-Educational Battery: Tests of Achievement

Reading	GE *3.0*	AE *8-2*	%ile *5*	SS *75*
Word Identification		Grade Range *2.5–3.5*		
Word Attack		Grade Range *2.3–3.0*		
Passage Comprehension		Grade Range *3.0–4.0*		
Mathematics	GE *3.8*	AE *9-0*	%ile *2*	SS *69*

Calculation	Grade Range *3.0–4.0*			
Applied Problems	Grade Range *3.0–4.0*			
Written Expression	GE *3.3*	AE *8-4*	%ile *1*	SS *65*
Dictation	Grade Range *2.5–3.5*			
Proofing	Grade Range *2.5–3.5*			
Punctuation and Capitalization	Grade Range *2.5–3.5*			
Spelling	Grade Range *2.5–3.5*			
Usage	Grade Range *2.5–3.5*			

Test of Written Language (TOWL): Written Language Quotient *65*

Vocabulary	%ile *9*	SS *80*
Thematic Maturity	%ile *2*	SS *69*
Spelling	%ile *2*	SS *69*
Word Usage	%ile *5*	SS *75*
Style	%ile *1*	SS *65*

Classroom Reading Inventory (Silvaroli): Listening Comprehension

Grade Level	*Comprehension*
2nd grade	*90%*
3rd grade	*80%*
4th grade	*75%*
5th grade	*75%*
6th grade	*45%*

Testing Interpretation

Learning Modality. Testing results indicate severely deficit functioning in perceptual processing skills for age and grade expectations, but commensurate with cognitive expectations unless a written product is required. Dallas's performance on the *Woodcock-Johnson* visual perceptual speed items revealed a high level of accuracy on visual matching of numerals (94%) at the 3rd to 5th grade range. He also performed at a high level of accuracy on spatial relations tasks (91% items, 90% puzzles) at the 4th to 6th grade range. On the *Slingerland,* Dallas was successful on visual memory (90%) and visual discrimination (86%) tasks. However, when visual memory was paired with a required written response, Dallas experienced significant difficulties with spelling and sequencing of items.

Dallas's performance on the *Woodcock-Johnson* auditory memory tasks at GE 4.4 was commensurate with cognitive expectations. Memory for sentences was good (4.0–5.0 grade range), but he experienced difficulty with auditory memory and reauditorization of numbers (3.0–4.0 grade range) which substantiated the *WAIS-R* performance on the Digit Span subtest. The *Slingerland* indicated good auditory discrimination skills (92%). When auditory memory was paired with a written response, Dallas experienced significant difficulties (56% items, 63% sequencing).

Reading and Listening Comprehension. Dallas's overall performance in reading indicates a severe weakness for age and grade expectations, but commensurate with cognitive expectations. Word attack and word identification skills at the 2.5–3.5 grade range indicated that he has not acquired basic sight vocabulary, and has not mastered basic phonic and structural analysis decoding skills. During oral reading he read word-by-word. Dallas attempted to use his minimal phonics skills, but they were not effective in decoding unknown words due to short vowel and consonant substitutions. Dallas's higher performance on reading comprehension (3.0–4.0 grade range) indicates that he is using context clues in deriving meaning from a passage.

Listening comprehension appears to be at the 5th grade instructional level. Dallas experienced difficulty with inference, evaluation, and drawing conclusions questions, while answering correctly questions regarding details and literal level information. He experienced difficulty defining words that were not specifically defined in context.

Mathematics. Dallas's overall performance in mathematics on the *Woodcock-Johnson* indicates severe deficits for age and grade expectations, but appears commensurate with cognitive expectations (GE 3.8). He committed at least five calculation errors due to lack of attention to the process sign, thus, performing the wrong process. He appears not to know the basic math facts as he used his fingers in calculation. Dallas appears to understand the algorithms of addition and subtraction with regrouping. He does not appear to understand the algorithms of multiplication and division. He did not attempt to calculate any problems involving fractions.

On the applied problems subtest, Dallas experienced difficulty with abstract calculation and problem-solving needing a visual picture of problems or computing on his fingers. He appears to understand the relationship concepts that indicate which mathematical process to use in problem-solving. Dallas experienced much difficulty in attempting to solve two-step problems. He, also, experienced difficulty sorting through extraneous information to isolate the critical information required to calculate the problem. Dallas had difficulty solving problems dealing with money, time, and measurement.

Written Expression. Dallas's overall performance on the *Woodcock-Johnson* in written expression indicates severe deficits for age and grade expectations, but appears commensurate with cognitive expectations (GE 3.3). His performance in knowledge of written expression rules of punctuation, capitalization, spelling, word usage, proofing appear to be in the 2.5–3.5 grade range. He experienced difficulty with irregularly formed plurals.

On the *TOWL*, Dallas experienced difficulty with verb tenses on the Word Usage subtest. Primary problems in Style included apostrophes, quotation marks, and commas. Deficits in spelling are significantly related to lack of skill mastery in phonics and structural analysis. Dallas's expressive story (creative writing sample) was analyzed for higher level vocabulary and appears to be above cognitive expectations. He appears to be functioning commensurate with cognitive expectations in thematic maturity in which he used two of the twenty thematic maturity evaluation items.

Informal assessment of the creative writing sample indicates an immature story response in story content and structure. Dallas did not write a complete story with a beginning, middle, and ending. He did not write in complete sentences, but he did write in complete simple thoughts. Dallas wrote primarily in run-on sentences connected by "and." He did not use his knowledge of capitalization and punctuation, inconsistently capitalizing nouns and omitting punctuation.

Summary. The auditory and visual modes of learning appear adequate with an oral or circled response. However, auditory and visual memory with a written response is a severe deficit area. Dallas lacks automaticity in handwriting, written expression mechanics (capitalization and punctuation), phonics and structural analysis, and fine motor coordination, which significantly interferes with all tasks requiring expressive writing.

Dallas appears to be functioning significantly below age and grade expectations, but commensurate with cognitive expectations in all academic areas with overall functioning in the 3rd to 4th grade range. Listening comprehension at the 5th grade level is a strength.

Educational Diagnostician

Social and Emotional Development (Informal Assessment)

Dallas is making progress in social and emotional development. He has attended a personal development class three times per week for 30 minutes each during the past academic year and this school year as well. The focus of this class is improving social development skills.

Social Perspective-Taking. Dallas experiences difficulty in social perspective-taking. He recognizes and shows concern about how others feel and expresses concern for others. Since he functions primarily at a literal level, he has difficulty making inferences about characteristics of people. He cannot anticipate how another's personality will affect his own behavior (social inferences). He understands at the literal level the reciprocal nature of social interactions, thus, engages in social comparison between himself and others.

Social Regulation and Moral Development. Dallas experiences difficulty in conforming to several sets of rules regarding moral codes and behaviors. He assumes certain roles based on the unrestrained responses of others. He is very much influenced by the behavior code that his father and male relatives espouse that "real men" work on cars, fix electrical things, and are involved in sports and hunting. Thus, Dallas is aware of some nuances of unwritten rules and codes of conduct.

Dallas's current understanding of the social world is quite limited and he does not learn easily through indirect socialization techniques. He participates in sports that involve public comparison and competition. Dallas is beginning to understand that appropriate behavior differs in various social settings. He is sensitive to the negative reactions of family and peers.

Social Problem-Solving. Dallas experiences difficulty in social problem solving, in academic problem-solving, and in problem-solving in other areas as well. Social problem-solving is more difficult because Dallas functions primarily on a literal or concrete level, experiences difficulty understanding cause and effect relationships, and experiences difficulty in understanding social perspective-taking and social regulation. Dallas experiences difficulty understanding social problems and social consequences. His problem-solving approach is primarily trial and error.

Social Relationships. Dallas does not appear to be experiencing emerging independence from parents and emotional conflicts between his peer group code and adult rules. In Dallas's social situation the men and boys "hang out" together with the men serving as role-models for the boys. Dallas interacts with peers in unsupervised situations, but most of his activities are directly or indirectly supervised. He has learned to avoid trouble by spending most of his free time "hanging around" the shop with family and friends. Dallas is quiet and rather shy. He has not learned the art of negotiation. He does not date, and is immature in social interpersonal relationships.

Summary. Dallas experiences difficulty with social inferences, social problem-solving, social regulation, social problems and consequences, negotiation, and interpersonal relationships. Dallas is a nice person, who is concerned about the feelings of others, and wants to get along harmoniously.

Guidance Counselor

Social Communication

Test Administered

Social Communication Skills for Handicapped Adolescents (pre/post tests)

Testing Interpretation

Dallas has attended a social communication class 3 times per week for 30 minutes since the past academic year. The lessons are frequently correlated with those of the social development class. The purpose is to enhance transitional skills.

Emotional and Body Language. Dallas has successfully completed the units on emotions and body language. He understands and recognizes the basic emotions (happy, sad, angry, afraid), and the appropriate way to express them. He understands facial, bodily, and verbal expressions of these emotions. He has improved significantly in interpreting his own feelings and those of others. He can read body language, and use body language and common gestures to communicate. Dallas understands the importance of avoiding intrusive body language such as inappropriate touching and talking in someone's face. He recognizes the role of vocal inflections in expressing feelings and uses the appropriate vocal inflection when delivering a message. Dallas understands that verbal and nonverbal messages must match or the person sends "mixed" messages.

Communication Styles and Conversation Skills. Dallas has successfully completed the units on communication styles and conversation skills. He understands the basic communication styles (passive, aggressive, assertive) and various aspects of facial expression, body posture, and tone of voice that are characteristic of each style. He recognizes his current style of communication, and can determine which style others are using. He has role played answering questions assertively using appropriate posture, voice, facial expressions; and preventing fear and anger from disrupting communication.

Dallas understands the basic conversation skills including listening strategies; speaker and listener rules; conversational rules of initiating, maintaining, and concluding a conversation. He also understands the proper ways to gain attention, and the pragmatically appropriate and inappropriate manner in making requests and asking for information.

Interpersonal Skills and Conflict Management Skills. Dallas has not as yet been introduced to the units on interpersonal and conflict management skills. Pretests indicated significant interpersonal skill deficits in behavior appropriate to the situation, appropriate ways to tease and to respond to teasing, dealing with embarrassment, and giving and receiving compliments. Pretests, also, indicated significant conflict management deficits in problem solving strategies, making and receiving complaints, giving and accepting constructive criticism, apologizing, dealing with false accusation, accepting consequences of behavior, and compromising.

Summary. Dallas has made significant improvement in social communication skills including interpreting and expressing emotions; using facial, body, and vocal expressions of emotions; recognizing and using basic communication styles; and understanding and using basic conversational skills. He experiences significant weaknesses in social communication and interpersonal skills, and social communication in conflict management.

Speech/Language Pathologist

Vocational Assessment

Informal Tests Administered

Informal Vocational Interest Survey	*Auto Mechanics*
Work Behaviors Simulations	*Satisfactory – Entry Level*

Competitive Employment Survival Skills	*Excellent*
Survival Vocabulary	*Satisfactory 85%*
Daily Living Simulations (and parent report)	
Self-Help Skills	*Mastered*
Consumer Skills	*Deficit*
Domestic Skills	*Satisfactory*
Health Care	*Satisfactory*
Knowledge of Community	*Satisfactory*

Testing Interpretation

Basic Academics. Reading assessment indicates that Dallas reads on the 3rd grade level. Current performance on the Survival Vocabulary test indicates that Dallas reads and understands 85% of the information signs, safety signs, employment signs (information and safety), transportation signs, community signs, medical words (hospital signs, symptoms, ailments, treatments), and grocery store words. He possesses functional reading skills.

Mathematics assessment indicates that Dallas is functioning on the 3rd grade level. He can add and subtract with regrouping, but cannot multiply or divide. He experienced significant difficulties in problem solving and with problems dealing with money, time, and measurement. Therefore, Dallas does not appear to possess survival and functional mathematics skills.

Verbal expressive and receptive language appear to be at the 3rd grade level. Speech and language appear to be adequate, but on a concrete level. Social communication class has improved his abilities in conversational skills. In written communication, Dallas appears to be functioning on a 3rd grade level, though he experiences difficulty with mechanics. He writes in complete simple thoughts, but not complete sentences.

Personal and Social Skills. Dallas appears to possess a positive self-concept. His emotional and personal adjustment appear satisfactory. The classes on personal development and social communication have helped significantly. He is weak in interpersonal skills and conflict management skills which need to continue to be part of his transition program.

Community Adjustment Skills. Dallas is completely independent in all self-help skills and in all his basic personal needs. He selects and color coordinates his own clothing, a skill that mother has emphasized at home.

Consumer skills are an area of weakness for Dallas. Since he works after school in his father's shop, parents have established his own checking account. He has the skills to balance his checkbook. He does not, however, have skills of budgeting and purchasing (e.g., getting the best deals).

In daily living simulations and home report from parents, Dallas has some kitchen skills. He can follow simple recipes, prepare boxed mixes, use the microwave oven to warm or cook, use the range top (electric) for cooking, and use the oven in baking. Though he does not like to, Dallas can adequately clean the kitchen and wash the dishes. At home he cleans his room and periodically helps vacuum the carpets. He is learning laundry and clothing care, and can iron his clothes. He can also sew on a button. Household management, maintenance, and repair are beyond his abilities as independent skills. However, he does mow the lawn and helps keep the yard and shop area cleaned when directed by parents.

Dallas has a basic understanding of health care. He understands the importance of a balanced diet. He has some basic first aid skills (e.g., cuts, burns, insect bites). He understands the importance of using over-the-counter drugs appropriately and following the directions. Dallas knows to dial 911 in case of a major accident or injury.

Dallas has a learner's permit and is taking driving lessons. Since they live in a small town where he has always lived, Dallas knows his way around town and the community expectations for his behavior. He knows how to use the telephone, and how and when to contact various emergency services (e.g., police, fire department).

Occupational Skills. Dallas accomplished 100% of the Competitive Employment Survival Skills which include basic academics, communication, personal and social skills, self-help skills, and work related behaviors. Currently, Dallas spends one-half day in an on-the-job training program at an auto service station. He follows directions appropriately, exhibits appropriate behavior at work, moves safely about the work place, asks co-workers when he needs help, works without disruptions when being observed, understands the importance of punctuality at work, stays on work task 1–2 hours if needed.

Auto mechanics is Dallas's vocational interest choice at present. In his on-the-job placement, he has learned some basics of routine auto servicing including changing the oil, checking the belts, patching a tire, checking various fluids, and putting a car on the rack. Dallas is making good progress in this placement.

Vocational Coordinator

Evaluation Summary

Dallas is a 16 year, 10 month old student who is currently enrolled in the Work Study Program. Current psychological evaluation indicates that he is functioning within the mildly mentally retarded range of intellectual functioning with little variability among verbal and psychomotor skills.

Academic functioning appears commensurate with cognitive expectations at the 3rd to 4th grade range. Auditory and visual modes of learning appear adequate unless a written response is required, then he functions in the severe deficit area. Dallas is functioning at the 3rd to 4th grade level in reading. Since he has not mastered phonics and structural analysis he has few decoding skills. In reading and listening comprehension (5th grade), Dallas easily answers literal level questions, but experiences significant difficulty with inferences. In math calculation, Dallas can add and subtract with regrouping, but cannot multiply or divide. He does not know basic math facts, and experiences significant difficulty with problem-solving, money, time, and measurement. Dallas experiences difficulty with written expression. He writes in complete thoughts, but not complete sentences omitting capitalization and punctuation.

In social development, Dallas experiences difficulty with social inferences, social problem-solving, social regulation, negotiation, and interpersonal relationships. In social communication, he can interpret and express emotions appropriately; use facial, body, and vocal expressions of emotions; recognize and use basic communication styles and conversation styles. He experiences difficulty with interpersonal communication skills and communication in conflict management.

Vocationally, Dallas is making good progress in his on-the-job placement at an auto service center. He scored 100% accuracy on the Competitive Employment Survival Skills. He possesses functional reading skills, but not functional math skills including consumer skills. His skills in self-help, domestic, health care, and knowledge of the community are satisfactory. Occupational skills appear to be quite good at the entry level in auto servicing. Dallas's performance on competitive employment skills indicated that he understands the expectations of himself as a worker.

Case Manager

DIAGNOSIS: Mildly Mentally Retarded

RE-EVALUATION REPORT
MARK

Age: 4 years, 8 months
Grade: Preschool for Multihandicapped Children
Date: May , 19___

Background and Educational Concerns

Reason for Referral

Mark is a 4 year, 8 month old student who attends a special preschool program for multihandicapped children. He has attended this program since he was two years old. Mark has numerous medical concerns as well as visual impairment and developmental delay in all areas. This is an Early Childhood Special Education re-evaluation for 5 year olds.

Health

School health records indicate that Mark receives clonopin for seizure disorder, and occasionally, dimetapp for allergies. His immunizations are current. Mark is nonambulatory and requires a wheelchair.

Medical records indicate that Mark experienced a post-operative cardiac arrest following corrective heart surgery as an infant which resulted in brain damage, vision impairment, convulsive disorders, neurological and motor control impairment.

Visual History

Medical examination at age two years indicated pale optic nerve heads. The following visual behaviors were noted: no corneal light reflex, fixated on white and red light, tracked red light to the right 45 degrees, sensory blink reflex present, direct and consensual pupillary reflexes present in left eye. Visual examination at age 3 years indicated the following visual behaviors: no protective blink reflex, no direct and consensual pupillary reflexes in right eye, no opticokinetic nystagmus, appeared to avoid light, no eye contact with persons or objects, no focus on objects.

Auditory History

Audiological testing at two years of age indicated normal tympanograms for both ears, behavioral responses to monitored live voice and noisemakers at 10–20 dB indicating normal hearing in at least one ear. At age three years, Mark's classroom teacher indicated that he responded to commands and speech in the classroom, was frightened by angry voices, recognized and responded to his name, stopped in response to "no", attended to music, and responded to speech by localizing.

Socio-Economic and Home Information

English is the language of the home. Mark lives with his mother and older sister, who attends Jr. High and cares for him after school. Mother, a registered nurse at the local hospital, works primarily day shifts. The family lives in a modest brick house in a stable working class neighborhood. The parents were divorced when Mark was about one year old. Father moved out-of-state and does not provide child support. Aid to Dependent Children and Social Rehabilitative Services contributes funds that help to offset Mark's medical expenses.

CURRENT MULTIDISCIPLINARY EVALUATION

This evaluation includes the following assessments: cognition, vision, hearing, communication, physical therapy, and social development.

Psychological Evaluation

Previous Test Administered

Battelle Developmental Inventory

CA *2 years, 4 months* MA *4–7 months*

Current Test Administered

The Callier-Azusa Scale (Cognition)

CA *4 years, 8 months* MA *18 months*

Testing Interpretation

Mark appears to be functioning at the 18 month level. He makes an effort to deliberately imitate sounds and movements of adults, vocalizes similar sounds in response to an adult, vocalizes babbling in response to an adult. Mark moves to regain an object moved out of his reach, searching with his hands. If the adult uses hand shaping, Mark will imitate the adult's movements. He performs consistent actions in response to familiar gestures (e.g., patting the table, shaking a toy). Mark uses causal action in a familiar game situation (e.g., pat-o-cake, tickling). He has integrated motor schemas such as banging objects on a table. He drops or throws objects. He will rotate some objects inspecting them, but usually inspects them by mouthing.

Mark realizes that objects continue to exist after he misplaces them and will search for them with his hand. He anticipates routine events from environmental cues. He imitates familiar gestures by gradual approximation and attempts to imitate complex gestures, generally he uses his left hand.

Mark demonstrates new schemas of playing through handshaping. He recognizes that other people can obtain an object or perform a task. He generally says, "go" when he wants something. Mark hears sounds from all sources. He says "go" when he wants an activity repeated. Mark will initiate a sequence of language exchanges, but not motor exchanges. Depending on behavior, he will imitate a new behavior without groping or error.

School Psychologist

School Vision Evaluation (Optometric Screening)

Previous ophthalmological evaluation at age 4 years indicated that Mark's eyes showed a full range of motion, but do not fix and follow large stimuli. His eyes were aligned and worked together signifying an image is being perceived by the brain and controlling their position. The optic nerve showed a mild paleness (minimal optic atrophy) probably related to the stoppage of blood flow to the brain during the cardiac arrest as an infant and further decreasing the vision. No other information was provided.

At this screening, Mark slowly moved his eyes in the direction of a penlight, flashlight, and transilluminated flashlight (red, yellow) when presented from his left, right, superior, and inferior. Responses were not consistent, and fixations were not central, steady or maintained. Mark occasionally made brief attempts to move his eyes in the direction of faces. He manifested a horizontal, large magnitude, low velocity nystagmus which was consistent. OKN was not elicited. Protective blink reflex was present.

It appears that Mark has light perception and light projection (moves eyes in direction of light presented). Since he does not make central, steady, and maintained fixations estimated corrected visual acuity may be 20/200 or less in the better eye. Mark manifested horizontal nystagmoid movements compatible with decreased visual acuity. Since visual acuity cannot be determined, it is difficult to determine if Mark falls into the category of legally blind or partially-sighted.

Optometrist

Hearing Evaluation

Tests Administered

Impedance Test
Behavioral Audiometry

Testing Interpretation

Previously, Mark has received four hearing evaluations at school. Since he will not tolerate earphones, his hearing is assessed by observing behavioral responses to various auditory stimuli presented in a sound field. Results have consistently indicated essentially normal hearing for at least one ear.

At this evaluation, Mark smiled, localized, or vocalized to various noisemakers in a sound-field at levels of 10 dB hearing level (HL) to 20 dB HL. Mark consistently responded to simple commands (e.g., "give kisses," "touch your nose") at 15 dB HL to 20 dB HL. Mark imitated familiar words/phrases (e.g., "Hey there, Mama," "Hi," "ball," "button," and "mama") at 15 dB HL. Impedance test for middle ear function has consistently shown normal middle ear function with both ears, and today's evaluation revealed the same results.

In summary, Mark's hearing is essentially normal for at least one ear. His behavioral responses in the test situation and classroom appear to be at or above expectations for his overall developmental level.

Educational Audiologist

Speech/Language Evaluation (Informal Assessment)

Mark appears to be functioning expressively at the 18 months level. At school he is using the following words and phrases meaningfully: go, me go, Mama, bye-bye, hi, ball, (bi pa) for diaper, potty, more, (ba ba) for drink. Currently, Mark independently babbles almost constantly incorporating a greater variety of sounds into his babbling which has begun to take on a sentence-like pattern. Mark perseverates on several words and phrases especially "tickle ball mama". During imitation games he sometimes appears to be attempting to imitate and then perseverates rather than imitates. He continues to shake his head "no," usually at meals. Mark says "more" when he wants more of an activity that he is enjoying or more to eat. He has begun to make up repetitive play games with himself (e.g., he does an action, says "go," and then repeats the action).

Receptively, Mark appears to be functioning at the 12–18 month level. If you ask, "What does Santa Claus say?" Mark will respond, "Ha, Ha, Ha." He will touch his nose, belly, and diaper when asked, "Where is your ________?" He is able to follow some simple verbal commands involving motor movement such as "roll over," "clap your hands," and "so big." He recognizes and responds to his own name. Mark will respond with excitement when asked, "Do you want to play *Beat It* or *Ghostbusters?*" He imitates the following words and phrases: tickle, my ball, papa, button, drink, butterfly, Michael, bubblegum; I'm a big guy; Hey there, Mama. At times these words and phrases emerge during babbling and are occasionally preceded by "I say."

Speech/Language Pathologist

Motor Evaluation

Tests Administered

Chart of Normal Development Informal Observation
Brigance Diagnostic Inventory of Early Development

Testing Interpretation

Gross Motor Skills. Mark's muscle tone in extremities is mildly hypertonic, right greater than left side. His trunk is hypotonic. Mark tends to fix in low back to maintain his balance in higher developmental skills (e.g., sitting, supported kneeling, supported standing), but he is not locked into this pattern. He has decreased rotation in the thorax supine. Improvements have been noted in muscle strength and coordination including (1) increased bearing of upper extremities in all-4's on belly crawls and when assisted from prone to sitting; (2) increased balance in sitting, supported on all-4's, and 1/2 kneeling; (3) increased rotation of trunk in supine, prone, sitting; (4) increased weight shift in sitting, assisted all-4's and 1/2 kneel to stand.

Mark sits independently tailor-fashion for 10–15 minute intervals with occasional upper extremities' protective extension. He needs assistance during standing to prevent falls. Mark rolls by flexing legs, rotating head, then pelvis. When balance reactions are tested in sitting, Mark shows decreased use of abdominals with decreased trunk rotation causing him to quickly go into protective responses. He is able to maintain supported standing with knees flexed for a few seconds but then relies on locked knees for support. Gross motor skills appear to be at the 7–9 months developmental level.

Fine Motor Skills. Mark's left hand is dominant. He has greatly increased the use of his right hand, so that now he is using both hands to interact with toys and to explore parts of his body. He continues to have decreased stability/weight shift of shoulder/scapula area. He primarily shifts weight better to the right (weight on elbow) while prone on elbows allowing him to reach with his left hand. He continues to chew and bang hands, left greater than right. Improvements in strength and coordination seem evident in the following areas: (1) increased weight bearing of both upper extremities, (2) increased reaching over head with both upper extremities, (3) radial palmar grasp on left with increased manipulation skills (emerging 3-jaw chuck), (4) ulnar palmar grasp on right. Mark readily takes objects out of a can and is increasing time holding onto preferred objects with left hand. Fine motor skills appear to be at the 10–12 months developmental level.

Self-Help Skills: Feeding. Mark now sits at the table for feeding. He independently reaches for his spoon and picks it up with his left hand. He will tolerate manipulation to scoop his food, but does not attempt any independent scooping. He independently brings his spoon to his mouth and returns it to the table. Mark finger feeds independently. He will search for the food with his right hand, though he predominantly relies on the left. He uses a left radial palmar grasp to bring food to his mouth. Mark picks up his cup and drinks from the rim. He is beginning to return the cup to the table, usually with a tactile cue. Feeding skills appear to be at the 12 months level.

Self-Help Skills: Dressing. Mark independently removes his socks and shoes. He assists in removing left arm from his coat and then will remove his right arm independently with a verbal cue. After assisting in removing left arm from pullover shirt, Mark will independently remove shirt from head and right arm. After both arms are placed in the sleeves of a T-shirt, Mark will put a T-shirt on over his head with physical assistance. Dressing skills appear to be at the 12 months developmental level.

Self-Help Skills: Toileting. Mark wears diapers at home, but he has begun wearing training pants at school. He sits on an adaptive toilet with a tray about 5 times per day for no more than 10 minute intervals. On an average day, he will urinate in the potty two times, but will still have wet pants on an average of 1–2 times a day.

Physical Therapist

Home Social Behavior

Test Administered

The Callier-Azusa Scale (Social Development)

CA *4 years, 8 months* Social Development *10–12 months*

Testing Interpretation

Mark's *Interactions With Adults* appear to be at the 10–12 months developmental level. He responds to person-to-person contact. When someone picks him up he puts his head on their shoulder and pats their back. He attends to adults' voices and responds by vocalizing. Mark differentiates familiar and unfamiliar adults. He is able to play a game such as pat-a-cake if the adult paces and maintains the game. He attempts to maintain contact with familiar adults when they start to leave. He actively seeks to sustain interactions by saying "go" or "more" to continue playing.

Mark responds to simple commands such as "no" by crying because he does not like correction.

On *Interactions With Environment,* Mark appears to be functioning at approximately the 10–12 month level. He shows an awareness of the presence or absence of sound, light, and tactile stimulation. He has a preferred eating schedule and shows preferences for particular foods. Mark exhibits different vocalizations and shows discomfort when hungry, wet, or in pain. He is aware of body movements and body parts, and moves and changes positions. He differentiates familiar and unfamiliar environments and responds to noticeable changes in familiar environments. Mark anticipates a familiar event in the presence of cues. He seeks his musical teddy bear for comfort in a stressful situation or when tired.

Mark's *Interactions With Other Children* appear to be at the 8 months developmental level. He shows awareness of other children, responds to other children's presence, and smiles and vocalizes to other children's voices. He attempts to initiate interactions with other children and responds to other children's attempts to interact.

Educational Diagnostician; Respondent: Mother

Evaluation Summary

Mark is a 4 year, 8 month old student currently attending a preschool for multihandicapped children. Mark appears to be functioning at the following levels:

Developmental Skill	*Level*
Cognition	18 months
Receptive language	12–18 months
Expressive language	18 months
Fine motor	10–12 months
Gross motor	7–9 months
Feeding and dressing	12 months
Toileting	6–9 months
Home social behavior	10–12 months

Mark has a chronic visual condition that has interfered with his visual learning mode. Fixations were not central, steady, or maintained. Opticokinetic nystagmus was not elicited. It appears that Mark has light perception and projection. Estimated corrected visual acuity may be 20/200 or less in the better eye. Mark manifested horizontal nystagmoid movements compatible with decreased visual acuity.

Mark has been seen on four occasions for hearing evaluations at school. The results have consistently indicated essentially normal hearing for at least one ear. He smiled, localized, or vocalized to various noisemakers in a sound field at levels of 10 dB to 20 dB hearing level. Impedance test for middle ear function has consistently shown normal middle ear function for both ears. Mark's observed behavioral responses in the test situation and classroom appear to be at or above expectations for his overall developmental level.

In the classroom, Mark meaningfully uses at least twenty words. He independently babbles constantly incorporating a greater variety of sounds. Muscle tone in extremities is mildly hypertonic and trunk is hypotonic. Improvements have been noted in muscle strength and coordination and increase in balance in sitting. Mark's left hand is dominant with a radial palmar grasp and emerging 3-jaw chuck.

Mark has a medical diagnosis of neurological impairment and impaired motor control as a result of post-operative cardiac arrest with brain damage.

Case Manager

DIAGNOSIS: Multihandicapped (visually impaired, moderately mentally retarded, and physically impaired)

RE-EVALUATION REPORT
VICKY

Age: 12 years, 10 months
Grade: Intermediate Moderately Retarded Program
Date: May , 19____

Background and Educational Concerns

Reason for Referral

Vicky is a 12 year, 10 month old student attending a self-contained intermediate level program for moderately mentally retarded students. She was initially diagnosed at 3 years of age at a Child Find Clinic and has received special education services for the past nine years. This evaluation was requested by her teacher to consider a possible placement change from the intermediate program in the elementary school to the program at the Junior High school.

Health: Immunizations are current. No current medical concerns were noted.

Vision and Hearing Screenings: Normal Range Acuities

Speech and Language Screenings

Speech and language appear appropriate for cognitive expectations.

Socio-Economic and Home Information

English is the language of the home. Vicky's father is an electrician and her mother works as a dental assistant. Vicky is the middle child, with an older and a younger sister, who are nonhandicapped. The family lives in a townhouse complex with other working class families. There is a park, recreation center, and swimming pool for after school and weekend activities. There appears to be no economic deprivation.

CURRENT MULTIDISCIPLINARY EVALUATION

This evaluation includes assessments in the following areas: intelligence, perception and memory, academic achievement, language, adaptive behavior, and social skills.

Psychological Evaluation

Test Administered

Wechsler Intelligence Scale for Children-Revised (WISC–R)

Verbal IQ	*46*	Performance IQ	*45*	Full Scale IQ	*45*
Information	*1*	Picture Completion	*4*		
Similarities	*3*	Picture Arrangement	*1*		
Arithmetic	*1*	Block Design	*1*		
Vocabulary	*1*	Object Assembly	*1*		
Comprehension	*1*	Coding	*1*		
Digit Span	*1*				

Testing Interpretation

Vicky is a 12 year, 10 months old student attending a self-contained class for moderately retarded students. She came to the testing very shyly and initially responded so softly to questions that her voice was barely audible. With much verbal praise and light teasing, she relaxed and responded appropriately.

Current results of the *WISC–R* indicate functioning within the moderate retardation range, as indicated in past assessment, with little variability among verbal expressive and psychomotor abilities. There are no significant strengths indicated in this assessment. Relative strengths in verbal expressive abilities at the upper limits of retardation were noted in concrete kinds of thinking and verbal concept formation. Relative strengths in psychomotor abilities at the lower limits of the borderline range were noted in ability to recognize essential details in pictures.

In summary, Vicky's overall cognitive functioning lies within the moderate range of intelligence (*FSIQ 45*) with no significant discrepancies.

School Psychologist

Psycho-Educational Evaluation

Tests Administered

Woodcock-Johnson Psycho-Educational Battery: Tests of Achievement

Reading	GE 1.9	AE 7-1	%ile <1	SS <65
Mathematics	GE 1.0	AE 5-10	%ile <1	SS <65
Written Expression	GE 1.1	AE 6-1	%ile <1	SS <65

Slingerland Screening Test, Form A

Far Point Copying	*Good*
Near Point Copying	*Good*
Visual Memory	*80%*
Visual Discrimination	*100%*
Visual Memory/Written Response	*70%*
Auditory Memory/Written Response	*40%*
Auditory Discrimination	*70%*

Woodcock-Johnson Psycho-Educational Battery: Tests of Cognitive Ability

Visual Perceptual Speed	GE *1.0*	AE *5-10*	%ile <*1*	SS <*65*
Visual Matching (80%)		Grade Range *1.0*		
Spatial Relations (96%)		Grade Range *1.0*		
Auditory Memory Cluster	GE *1.0*	AE *4-8*	%ile <*1*	SS <*65*
Memory for Sentences		Grade Range *1.0*		
Numbers Reversed		Grade Range *1.0*		

Brigance Diagnostic Inventory of Basic Skills: Math Readiness

Skills Within (+), Below (−) Age/Grade Expectancy

Counting to 39	−
Numeral Recognition to 10	−
Writing Numbers to 10	−
Counting Objects to 10	−
Joining Sets	−
Ordinal Concepts	−

Classroom Reading Inventory (Silvaroli): Forms A and B

Level	Word Recognition	Reading Comprehension	Listening Comprehension
1	95%	90%	90%
2	75%	60%	50%
3	40%	0%	0%

Testing Interpretation

Learning Modality. Testing indicates that Vicky's visual learning channel is significantly stronger than the auditory channel. On the *Woodcock-Johnson,* she performed significantly below age and grade expectations and similar to that of a kindergarten student aged 5 years,

10 months. On the visual matching of numerals task, she correctly responded to 80% of the items attempted experiencing several number transpositions. On the spatial relations task, Vicky correctly responded to 90% of the items attempted. Performance of visual perceptual tasks on the *Slingerland* (1st to 2nd grade level) indicated good visual discrimination (100%), visual memory (80%), and visual memory with a written response (70%).

Testing indicates significantly weak auditory learning skills. On the *Woodcock-Johnson,* Vicky's performance was similar to that of a child aged 4 years, 10 months, which is significantly below age, grade, and cognitive expectations. She accurately remembered and repeated six-word sentences. Vicky did not understand the task required of her on the numbers reversed (auditory reorganization) subtest. Despite numerous examples, she could not accurately reverse a two digit number. On the *Slingerland,* Vicky experienced considerable difficulty with auditory discrimination (50%) and auditory memory with a written response (40%).

Reading and Listening Comprehension. Reading appears to be an area of strength for Vicky with performance at GE 1.9 on the *Woodcock-Johnson* in word recognition, word attack, and passage comprehension. Vicky recognizes words with both upper and lower case letters at the beginning, knows the alphabet letters in sequence, and identifies words found in preprimers and primers. She knows some antonyms and some synonyms, and answers some "wh" questions. Word attack skills include naming initial consonants and initial digraphs, recognizing short vowels in one syllable words, recognizing word endings, recognizing rhyming words and compound words. On the *Silvaroli* Vicky read orally in a monotone voice and primarily responded to fact questions. Her overall performance in reading at 1st grade instructional level indicated functioning significantly below expectations for age and grade expectations, but commensurate with cognitive expectations.

Performance in listening comprehension at the 1st grade instructional level was commensurate with cognitive expectations. Vicky appears to function primarily at the literal level and has great difficulty with inference and evaluation questions. In overall reading and listening comprehension, Vicky is functioning six years below age expectations, but commensurate with cognitive expectations.

Mathematics. Overall performance in mathematics on the *Woodcock-Johnson* indicates significantly deficit functioning (6–7 years deficit) at the kindergarten level. Vicky correctly answered three of the seven problems dealing with basic facts sums less than ten. Her performance on the applied problems subtest indicated that she does not understand the concepts of addition and subtraction. On the *Brigance,* Vicky could answer simple questions relating to one-to-one correspondence to 5; counts orally to 10, writes 0–5, and identifies 0–5; solves oral problems using "one more" or "one less"; recognizes, matches, and reproduces circles, squares, and triangles; divides shapes in half.

Written Expression. On the *Woodcock-Johnson,* Vicky's overall performance in written expression indicated functioning at the beginning of 1st grade level. She correctly wrote upper and lower case letters on the spelling test, but spelled no words correctly. Informal assessment indicates that Vicky spells her own 1st and last names; a few one syllable phonetic words such as "cat." On the proofing subtest, she recognized one capitalization error. Vicky's knowledge of capitalization and punctuation is limited primarily to knowledge that sentences begin with a capital letter and end with a period. On the *Slingerland,* copying exercises indicated adequate manuscript handwriting. She wrote slowly and copied one letter at a time. Lack of automaticity in written language mechanics precludes written composition.

Summary. Vicky's performance indicates that the visual modality is her strongest for learning with an oral or written response. Visual perceptual skills appear to be at the kindergarten to 1st grade functioning level. Auditory perceptual skills at preschool functioning ability are a severe deficit for age, grade, and cognitive expectations. Auditory memory for words and numbers are both significantly deficit.

Academically, Vicky is functioning 6–7 years deficit for age and grade expectations. Reading and listening appear commensurate to above cognitive expectations, while mathematics and written expression are deficit even for cognitive expectations.

Educational Diagnostician

Speech and Language Evaluation

Tests Administered

Language Screening Sample (Informal)
Northwest Syntax Screening Test (NSST)
Informal Articulation Test

Testing Interpretation

Receptive and Expressive Language. Vicky's performance on the *NSST* indicates functioning at the 6–7 year level in expressive and receptive language. Informal language screening indicates that Vicky has acquired simple plurals, verbs (past, present, future tense), possessives, personal pronouns, and prepositions (e.g., over, under, after, before, into, down, near), and simple comparatives. Emerging skills include understanding "if" and "because." She has difficulty with simple analogies. Vicky reads on a preprimer level, can use a picture dictionary, and defines and explains words. She asks questions and follows simple directions.

Pragmatics. Pragmatics are rather difficult for Vicky as she is shy. She understands that communication is an exchange of greetings or information. She experiences difficulty in interpreting facial and body language and vocal intonation. A major focus in language class this academic year was initiating and ending conversations with teachers and other students. She speaks primarily in simple concrete sentences.

Speech. Informal assessment indicates that Vicky is functioning on the 6–7 year level in speech skills. She correctly articulates most single consonants, blends, and digraphs. She still experiences difficulty with /y/, /th/, /z/, /s/, /kt/, /tr/, and /sp/. Voice, fluency, and oral peripheral structures are within normal limits.

Summary. Vicky appears to be functioning at the 6–7 year level in receptive and expressive language, speech, and pragmatics. She continues to experience difficulty with nonlinguistic aspects of communication.

Speech/Language Pathologist

Adaptive Behavior

Tests Administered

Vineland Social Maturity Scale AE *6 years, 2 months*
Informal Teacher Assessment

Testing Interpretation

Self-Help Skills. Vicky is independent in eating, toileting, dressing, and grooming skills. She serves herself at the table, uses the utensils correctly, eats with her mouth closed, and behaves appropriately. She selects her own clothes (color coordinated) to wear to school; buttons, ties, snaps, and zips. Grooming is independent: bathing, washing hair and blow drying, keeping neat. These skills are a continuous focus at home and at school.

Daily Living Skills. Vicky enjoys helping mother around the house and has learned a number of skills at school. She can wash and dry dishes, but has difficulty with pots and pans. She is learning to load and operate the dishwasher. She can operate kitchen appliances such as the toaster and blender. She can heat simple dishes in the microwave oven. She is learning to cook simple dishes, make snacks, and follow simple recipes. She enjoys cooking (under supervision). Vicky can set and clear the table, and sweep the floor. She has difficulty operating the washing machine, but operates the clothes dryer and folds and puts clothes away when dry. Vicky can iron flat items (e.g., table cloth) and simple constructed garments.

Classroom Skills. Vicky listens and follows directions. Since her auditory skills are weaker than visual, it is helpful to pair oral directions with a visual or actual demonstration. She is very conscientious and wants to please. Vicky will continue to work on a task until completed. She puts away supplies that she has gotten out to work on a project. She especially enjoys cutting, pasting, coloring, and making art "things." Vicky is responsible and can be sent to the office on an errand (e.g., deliver attendance sheet) and return in a reasonable time. She does not interrupt classmates when they are working.

When asked to modify her behavior (e.g., talk softly, stay in your seat), Vicky complies without back-talk and grumbling. She participates in group activities even on new skills or in areas which she knows she can not do well. She understands classroom rules. She behaves appropriately in the halls, bathroom, and lunchroom.

Vicky is learning to use the computer to study vocabulary words and complete assignments. She enjoys computer games. She is proud of the new things she is learning to do and thrives on frequent praise.

Community Skills. Vicky is learning the value of money and how to use money in purchasing items. She cannot make correct change or give correct amounts for a purchase if change is required. She behaves appropriately on the school bus. She cannot use the city transportation system to go places, but she can go to the corner grocery store and purchase a loaf of bread for mother.

Vicky belongs to Girl Scouts and participates in church and social activities. She, also, attends the activities of her sisters. During the summer she takes swimming lessons.

Summary. Vicky's adaptive behavior appears commensurate with cognitive expectations. Often she will function above expectations due to high motivation, and family assistance and encouragement.

School Counselor

Evaluation Summary

Vicky is a 12 year, 10 month old student currently enrolled in a self-contained intermediate program for moderately retarded students. Current psychological evaluation indicates overall cognitive functioning within the moderate range of intelligence (FS IQ 45) with little variability among verbal expressive and psychomotor skills. Visual perceptual skills (kindergarten level) appear significantly stronger than auditory perceptual skills (preschool level). Performance is better with an oral or circled response than written response.

Academically, Vicky is functioning approximately six years deficit for age expectations. Her strongest area appears to be reading at GE 1.9. Oral reading and listening comprehension are at 1st grade instructional level. Mathematics is an area of significant deficit even for cognitive expectations with functioning at early kindergarten level. She experiences difficulty with all math readiness tasks and appears not to understand the concepts of addition and subtraction. Written expression at GE 1.1 is weak for cognitive expectations, however, the lack of automaticity in written expression prerequisites inhibits creative fluency.

Speech and language skills appear appropriate for cognitive expectations. Vicky continues to experience difficulty with the nonlinguistic aspects of pragmatics.

Adaptive behavior in self-help skills, daily living skills, classroom and community skills appear appropriate to cognitive expectations. She appears to be a pleasant, easy-going, highly motivated student.

Case Manager

DIAGNOSIS: Moderately Mentally Retarded

RE-EVALUATION REPORT
SAM

Age: 14 years, 6 months
Grade: Ungraded Adolescent Program for Deaf-Blind
Date: May , 19___

Background and Educational Concerns

Reason for Referral

Sam is a 14 year, 6 months old student attending an ungraded adolescent deaf-blind program at Washington Special School. Sam's original evaluation in Kentucky at age 9 years, 6 months resulted in a diagnosis of deaf-blind. Sam transferred to Washington School District three years ago and was enrolled in a special day school, self-contained class for deaf-blind students. Sam is receiving deaf-blind programming, indirect physical therapy, and indirect speech therapy services. This is a routine three year re-evaluation.

Health

School health records indicate that Sam receives no medication. He has a heart murmur, but no other outstanding medical concerns at this time. Sam's immunizations are current. He does not have orthopedic involvement nor requires personal or building modifications.

Medical records indicate a history of vision and hearing handicaps secondary to maternal rubella. At six months of age Sam had surgery to correct a heart valve that did not close. At ages fifteen months and eighteen months, he had surgery to remove cataracts on both eyes.

Vision History

An evaluation one year ago indicated that Sam manifests some of the ocular signs commonly seen in children affected by congenital rubella syndrome. Sam wears aphakic soft contact lenses corrected to 20/200. He reads large print and numbers at a distance of 1–4 inches. During the evaluation last year the following visual behaviors were noted: fixated with each eye separately, tracked with each eye in all directions, recognized known individuals by sight, completed school tasks 4–6 inches from face, and recognized a 1/8″ dot at 8″ from the face.

Auditory History

A hearing evaluation 2 years ago indicated moderately severe sensorineural hearing loss in both ears. Audiological testing one year ago indicated that pure tone air conduction thresholds showed a severe to profound hearing loss in the right ear and a severe hearing loss in the left ear. Sam, also, had bilateral myringotomies with tubes. Several months after the auditory testing, additional audiological testing was conducted in order to make a judgment regarding hearing aid purchase. With the Danavox aid he responded at the 25 dB level. During audiological testing toward the end of May with the Danavox 125-1, PPAGC hearing aid fit to the right ear, Sam responded to 30dB level. He receives good benefit from his hearing aid.

Socio-Economic and Home Information

English is the language of the home. Sam's father is plant manager at a local cosmetic manufacturing plant, and his mother is the children's librarian at the public library. Sam has a younger sister, Ellen, who is in the 5th grade. The family lives in a middle class suburban neighborhood. There appears to be no economic disadvantage.

CURRENT MULTIDISCIPLINARY EVALUATION

This evaluation includes the following assessments: cognition, vision, hearing, communication, motor skills, academic skills, and adaptive behavior.

Psychological Evaluation

Previous Tests Administered

Leiter International Performance Scale	CA *9-2*	MA *5-6*	IQ *58*
The Hiskey-Nebraska Test of Learning Aptitude	CA *9-2*	LA *5-0*	IQ *52.6*

Current Tests Administered

Perkins-Binet Intelligence Scale for the Blind	CA *14-6*	MA *6-10*
Leiter International Performance Scale	CA *14-6*	MA *6-8*

Testing Interpretation

Sam was a cooperative young man who seemed occasionally frustrated by his lack of ability to communicate. He uses signing and vocal approximations to communicate. When working with test materials he must look very closely at them. Medical records indicate a severe bilateral hearing loss for which he wears aids, and a significant visual impairment for which he wears glasses. Task persistence was fairly good. Sam was rapid in his work, but occasionally noticed his errors and self-corrected. His task focus was excellent, and when praised he would smile.

The *Perkins-Binet* was finally discontinued due to difficulties in communicating. Sam can answer simple comprehension questions and give simple definitions. However, more complex questions requiring thought abstraction were too difficult. Sam does best when the answer can be made associatively (e.g., "What do we use keys for?" rather than "What is a key?"). He has simple math concepts of direct counting, can recite the days of the week, make analogies at the year VII level, copy bead chain designs, and copy simple block designs. Testing on the *Perkins* suggests overall functioning is around the 6 year, 10 months level with skills continuing up through the year IX level.

On the *Leiter,* Sam performed at a 6 year, 8 months level with skills noted up through year VIII. He did well when directly matching block designs, shades of gray, and by genus. He could also complete a pattern and sequence designs for the circle series and the radii series. Difficulty was noted with more abstract tasks such as matching clothing, items by use, analogous designs, mass, or finely discriminated items such as footprints, dot estimation or mass. He did not understand line completion, concealed cubes, or the necessity of alignment in block designs. Visual difficulties undoubtedly interfered significantly with some of these tasks, but poor conceptual development enabling Sam to move from the concrete to abstract thought processes also interfered.

In summary, Sam appears to function within the moderately mentally retarded range of intelligence. However, due to the multiplicity of his sensory handicaps, this must be regarded as only a minimal estimate of his true potential. It is the opinion of this examiner that while some retardation is probably present, the current scores are depressed. Therefore, results of psychometric assessment should be interpreted with great caution.

School Psychologist

Vision Evaluation (Optometric Screening)

Previous Optometric examination last year indicated bilateral aphakia corrected with soft daily wear contact lenses. Sam's best corrected visual acuity has not been recorded better than 20/200 from either eye.

Current assessment indicates with contact lenses in place both visual acuities were measured at the following levels: OD (right) 20/200 Snellen letter recognized at 7 feet, a 20/100 letter was seen at 3–3½ feet; OS (left) 20/200 Snellen letter recognized at 2 feet. The right visual acuity at near was 20/70 reduced Snellen letter or a number recognized at 3–4 inches. It seemed as if all of Sam's near visual tasks were completed at a working distance proportional to the size of the print or task.

OD (right) fixation was fairly central, but not steady or easily maintained. OS (left) fixational ability was poor. OD tracking was rough in all directions. No tracking ability was apparent OS. Sam manifested an alternating esotropia, however, had strong preference for the OD which measured better visual acuity. He manifested a constant, moderate velocity, moderate magnitude horizontal nystagmus. Sam appears to fall within the legally blind status.

Optometrist

Hearing Evaluation

Tests Administered

Impedance Testing
Electroacoustic Analysis of Hearing Aids and Tolerance Testing
Behavioral Audiometry

Testing Interpretation

Impedance test for middle ear function shows normal tympanograms. Tolerance testing revealed that Sam is able to tolerate 123 dB SPL in both ears. He uses binaural Danavox 125 PP AGC hearing aids. An electroacoustic analysis of the hearing aids indicated they were functioning properly. A hearing aid evaluation in the sound field yielded the following results:

Hearing Aid: Danavox 136 PP AGC			Volume Control
Right Ear	#ER5083	Setting: PO/G–O/H-12/A-65	6
Left Ear	#P4345	P-10/G-10/H–O/A-85	6

Aided Ear	Speech Threshold	5% Warble Tones 500	1K	2K	4K	8K
Right	30 dB	55	35	40	50	NR
Left	20 dB	40	35	40	55	NR

Pure tone air conduction thresholds show a severe hearing loss in both ears. Results on this annual hearing evaluation are similar to those found on previous hearing evaluations. Sam receives good benefit from his hearing aids.

Educational Audiologist

Communication Evaluation (Informal Assessment)

Speech

Sam communicates through Total Communication, consistently vocalizing while signing. He uses his residual hearing well and appears to rely upon his hearing for receptive communication. He imitates normal stress patterns of speech. Due to poor fine motor control and poor motor planning, Sam has been unable to coordinate intelligible speech with signing. He can correctly articulate a few words during intensive speech drill, but there has been no carry over. Sam appears frustrated during speech drill.

Language

In structured situations, Sam is able to describe action pictures in 3–5 word sentences using English structures including the article "the," the verb "is," nouns, verbs, prepositions, and adjectives. Occasionally, he reverts to ASL. Sam is able to answer a large variety of questions (e.g., who, what, where, when in connection with calendar, how many, do you ______, etc.) appropriately. He asks questions mainly through voice inflection and facial expression (lunch?, sick?, angry?) and asks permission to leave the room ("Bathroom, please? Water, please?"). He generally does not ask questions to gain new information but rather to confirm his own observations. In structured language sessions designed to teach Sam the skill of asking the questions "who" and "where," Sam models the question and answers it himself. He does not yet differentiate the role of the sender and the receiver. Sam directs the majority of his communication to adults. Language interaction with peers must be modeled or prompted.

Speech/Language Pathologist

Motor and Posture Evaluation (Informal Assessment)

Sam has rounded shoulders. There are contractures in his shoulders bilateral (flexion −20 and internal rotation 15 degrees). These limits on his range do not impair him functionally, but prevent his assuming pivot prone or standing back flat against the wall. Balance and equilibrium reactions are good. Visual-gross motor tasks are difficult for Sam including walking on a balance beam, tossing a ball, performing skipping or hopping patterns and moving contralateral extremities. He has good manual dexterity, prefers left hand. Visual-fine motor tasks are problematic. Sam does not cross the midline, does not correct shapes when copying, and does not order shapes in patterns if required by the task.

Physical Therapist

Academic Evaluation (Informal Assessment)

Reading and Listening Skills

Informal testing indicates reading functioning at approximately the 1st grade level. Sam recognizes color and number words (1–10), names of family members, classmates and staff with 100% accuracy and selected words (chosen on the basis of classroom activities) with 70% accuracy. He is learning some survival vocabulary including Grocery Store Words, Survival Words, and Safety Signs (words and phrases). Sam is learning to read by the whole word method. He has no decoding skills. He enjoys reading picture books with very short sentences and lots of activity in the pictures.

Listening comprehension appears to be at the 1st to 2nd grade level. Sam enjoys listening to tapes of illustrated high interest-low vocabulary books with most of the activity in the pictures. He primarily answers fact questions. Sam experiences great difficulty answering main idea, sequencing events, and cause-effect questions.

Mathematics. Sam appears to be functioning on the 2nd grade level in addition and subtraction calculation. Sam loves to work with numbers and actively seeks out tasks in this area. He is able to sign numbers 0–100, complete number sequences (e.g., 10, 11, ______, ______, ______, 15), and write numbers up to 200. He is able to complete simple addition and subtraction problems of any amount, though, he sometimes needs to be reminded to complete the columns of numbers from right to left. He is able to solve addition problems involving carrying with supervision. Sam makes use of his fingers or "counting upwards" mentally to solve subtraction problems through 20 that necessitate borrowing. Sam can measure objects under 12″ to the inch, and tell time on the hour. He has little concept of money; and no concept of multiplication, division, fractions, story problems.

Written Language

Sam can write his first and last names. He does not have a spelling vocabulary and writing sentences has not been part of his programming. He has shown no interest in writing.

Prevocational Skills

Sam can complete a variety of pre-vocational tasks in the areas of sorting, packaging, and assembling with 95–100% accuracy. He works independently at a consistent rate with few, if any, work stoppages, and is highly motivated to increase his work output. Sam's rate varies between 25 to 50% of the standard industrial rate depending upon the operations needed to complete the task.

Special Education Classroom Teacher

Vocational Evaluation

Tests Administered

Competitive Employment Survival Skills (Informal Test)	*Deficit*
Vocational Interest Survey (Informal)	*No Preference*
Work Behaviors Simulations (Informal)	*Satisfactory*
Survival Vocabulary	*Deficit*
Informal Daily Living Simulations (and parent report)	
Self-Help Skills	*Mastered*
Consumer Skills	*Severely Deficit*
Domestic Skills	*Deficit*
Health Care	*Deficit*
Knowledge of Community	*Deficit*

Testing Interpretation

Academics. Sam's reading at 1st grade level and math calculation at 1st to 2nd grade level indicate that he does not possess functional skills in these areas. Both expressive and receptive communication are areas of significant weakness. He uses signing with some verbal representations to communicate, but is difficult to understand for those who do not know him well.

Community Adjustment. Self-Help Skills are an area of strength for Sam as he is completely independent in personal care. He selects his own clothing and is independent in getting ready for school or outings.

The whole area of consumer skills is difficult for Sam. He does not have a good concept of the value of money. He does know if someone gives him the correct change to put into the coke machine that he can get a coke. He does not have a good grasp on the concept of purchasing, although can certainly find items that he desires when taken to the store.

Sam is learning some domestic skills at school and at home. He can straighten up his room at home and put away his possessions. He frequently sets the table and carries food to put on the table after it has been prepared. He can make snacks including sandwiches and cool-aid. He cannot use the stove top, oven, or microwave. Sometimes he washes dishes. Sam can use the vacuum cleaner and dust furniture. He can sort laundry by color and folds clean clothes taken from the clothes dryer. He has not learned the operation of the washing machine or ironing clothes.

Household management and maintenance are beyond his abilities as independent skills.

Sam understands to seek help in an emergency by locating a teacher or calling 911 on the telephone. He does not understand basic health care or nutrition. He does know that cuts need washed before applying a band-aid.

Sam's knowledge of the community is very limited. Due to his cognitive and sensory impairments, he is not allowed unsupervised activities within the community. He has some idea of the jobs of policemen and firemen. He has minimal knowledge of telephone usage. He knows the various types of stores frequented by his parents (e.g., bakery, grocery store, hardware store) and church, library, and other frequently attended places. He could not travel to these independently. He does not have independent use of the city transportation system.

Occupational Skills

Sam has an unclear idea of the type of work he would like to do. This needs to be explored more fully in the Adolescent Pre-Vocational/ Vocational Program. He is learning some pre-vocational skills of sorting, packaging, and assembly in the classroom.

On the Competitive Employment Survival Skills assessment, Sam was able to recite his full name, address, and phone number; complete some basic addition problems; follow one instruction at a time; maintain proper grooming; understand work routine and appropriate work behavior; communicate basic needs such as pain, help, toileting. Communication is a significant weakness both oral and written. Sam cannot write 3–5 word sentences, independently regroup addition and subtraction, or count change. He requires frequent and continuous supervision.

Vocational Counselor

Adaptive Behavior Evaluation

Test Administered

AAMD Adaptive Behavior Scale

Testing Interpretation

Sam's adaptive behavior was evaluated using the *AAMD Adaptive Behavior Scale* and compared to TMR and EMR norms. Compared to same aged EMR students, Sam's behavior appears to be below expectations in the areas of physical development, economic activity, language development, and mannerisms. His behavior in pre-vocational activity, self-direction, and responsibility appear to be above expectation for an EMR student. Sam's functioning in the areas of physical development, economic activity, and language development are severely negatively impacted by his vision and hearing limitations.

Compared to same-aged TMR students, Sam's behavior appears to be below expectations in the area of physical development, mannerisms, and symptomatic behavior. Again, Sam's severe vision and hearing deficits negatively affect his physical development. In the areas of time and numbers, prevocational activity, self-direction and responsibility, Sam functions significantly better than expectations for TMR students.

Sam's behavior is generally appropriate at school. He has no problems in the areas of aggression, antisocial behavior, rebelliousness, trustworthiness, withdrawal, interpersonal manners, acceptability of vocal habits, and activity.

Educational Diagnostician

Home Adaptive Behavior (Informal Parent Observation)

Sam handles personal care completely by himself except for trimming his nails. He shampoos and blow dries his hair, shaves, and chooses clothing. He uses signs coupled with vocalizing in communicating with family, teenagers, and some adults in community activities. Sam has learned self-control and is much calmer and better behaved than in the past. He will tell if something he did was wrong. At home he is a self-starter; he always has a project going. He likes to show his projects and receive praise. He likes to spend his free time looking at photo albums, library books, medical TV shows, watering plants, climbing trees, and building things.

He takes excellent care of his hearing aids and contact lenses. He is more casual about objects that are not so essential. Sam is eager to please and comply with family rules. He backslides on teasing his sister. Sam complies with community rules, wears his seatbelt in the car and on the school bus, waits patiently in lines. Sam takes his lunch money to school in his wallet. He learned the hard way not to give it to anyone but the teacher. Sam interacts well with authority figures. He wants to do right and does not want authority figures to be angry with him. Sam has begun having a friend ride the bus home from school with him.

Sam seems to prefer interacting with "regular" kids. He has several opportunities to interact including Sunday school, neighborhood activities, Saturday morning ice skating.

Guidance Counselor; Respondent: Mother

Evaluation Summary

Sam is a 14 year, 6 months old student attending an ungraded deaf-blind adolescent program. Current psychological evaluation indicates that Sam is functioning within the moderately mentally retarded range of intelligence. However, due to multiplicity of his sensory handicaps, this must be regarded as only a minimal estimate of his true potential. Testing suggests functioning around the 6 year, 10 months level with skills continuing through the 9 year level.

Optometric examination indicated bilateral aphakia corrected with soft daily wear contact lenses. Current screening indicated visual acuity of 20/200 right eye and left eye. Right eye fixation was fairly central, but not steady or easily maintained, and left eye fixational ability was poor. Right tracking was rough in all directions, and there was no tracking with the left eye.

Hearing evaluation indicated that pure tone air conduction thresholds showed a severe hearing loss in both ears functioning in the 70dB–90dB HL range. Impedance test for middle ear function showed tympanograms with rounded compliance peaks for both ears. Tolerance testing revealed that Sam is able to tolerate 123dB SPL in both ears. Sam receives good benefits from his hearing aids at 20dB to 30dB SPL.

In the classroom, Sam makes good use of his vision for ambulation, self-help, pre-vocational, and academic skills. He has little difficulty reading primary size print and with effort can read some finer print. Sam recognizes color and number words, names of family members and classmates, and selected classroom words. He signs 0–100, completes number sequences, writes numbers to 200, and adds and subtracts with no regrouping.

Sam communicates through Total Communication, consistently vocalizing while signing. He is able to describe action pictures in 3–5 word sentences. He is able to answer a large variety of questions. He directs the majority of his communication to adults. Language interaction with peers must be modeled or prompted. Due to poor motor control and poor motor planning he is unable to coordinate intelligible speech with signing. He functions on a 1st grade level in reading and on the 1st to 2nd grade level in mathematics. He has no written expression skills.

Visual-motor tasks are difficult. Sam completes a variety of pre-vocational tasks independently, at a consistent rate, and with 95–100% accuracy at 25 to 50% industrial rate. Pre-vocational assessment indicates deficits in competitive employment survival skills, consumer skills, domestic skills, health care, knowledge of community, and vocational interest. He demonstrated strength in work behavior simulations and self-help skills.

Adaptive behavior measures and classroom functioning indicate Sam's behavior is generally appropriate at school. Compared to same-aged EMR peers, Sam's performance is below expectations in the areas of physical development, economic activity, language development, and mannerisms (all affected by visual and hearing deficits). His performance in prevocational activity, self-direction, and responsibility appear to be above expectations for typical EMR peers. Sam's adaptive and social behavior at home and in the community are appropriate.

Case Manager

DIAGNOSIS: Deaf-blind, moderately mentally retarded

RE-EVALUATION REPORT
JEFF

Age: 5 years, 4 months
Grade: Ungraded Preschool for Severely Handicapped Students
Date: May , 19___

Background and Educational Concerns

Reason for Referral

Jeff is a 5 year, 4 months old preschool student who has received special education services since diagnosed severely multihandicapped (hearing impaired, physically impaired, profoundly mentally retarded) at 3 years, 4 months of age. Jeff attends the Preschool Program for Severely Handicapped Children. His extreme tactile defensiveness has significantly interfered with his developmental progress. This is an Early Childhood Special Education re-evaluation for five year olds.

Health

School health records indicate that immunizations are current. Jeff receives phenobarbitol and tegretol at breakfast and dinner for a seizure disorder, but receives no medication at school. He is nonambulatory and requires a wheelchair for locomotion.

Medical records indicate a history of cerebral palsy (mixed), seizure disorder, quadriplegia, hearing impairment, and mental retardation. Tactile defensiveness and vestibular dysfunction has interfered with the development of fine motor and self-help skills, gross motor and locomotion skills, and sensorimotor stage cognitive development.

Vision History

On initial evaluation at school at age 3 years, 4 months the following visual behaviors were noted: alternate use of eyes, blinked to bright lights, fixated on audio/visual stimulus and faces, tracked red light horizontally and vertically, visually avoided eye contact, scanned room to follow people, reached for visual stimulus at 4″ to 6″ distance. End-of-Year Report at age 4 years, 4 months indicated that Jeff fixated binocularly for 2–3 seconds, alternated the use of his eyes, made eye contact with caregiver and specific objects (preferred people or pictures of faces to objects), visually followed people as they moved around the classroom, tried to avoid visual teacher-directed activities.

Auditory History

An Evoked Response Audiometry test at 2 years revealed moderate to severe sensorineural hearing loss for the left ear and severe mixed hearing loss in the right ear. Behavioral hearing testing at age 3 years, 4 months indicated unaided responses at 70dB to 90dB HL, and aided 60dB to 70dB HL. Jeff wore an Opticon P11P body level hearing aid with a bone conduction vibrator. Recently, he received myringotomies with tubes for treatment of middle ear problems. The End-of-Year Report at age 4 years, 4 months indicated that in the classroom, Jeff startles to loud noises, does not respond to speech, but attends to hands when signing.

Developmental History

At age 2 years, 6 months, Jeff was evaluated by the United Cerebral Palsy Association and at age 3 years, 4 months he was evaluated by the Child Find Diagnostic Clinic. The results of these evaluations are as follows:

Developmental Skills	*2 years, 6 months*	*3 years, 4 months*
Cognition	0–3 months	0–3 months
Fine Motor	0–1 month	0–1 month
Gross Motor	3–5 months	3–5 months
Receptive Language	0–3 months	1–3 months
Expressive Language	0–3 months	1–3 months
Self-Help Age (Feeding)		6 months
Social Age		3–5 months

Developmental evaluation indicates very slow progress, approximately at the rate of 0–2 months progress per year.

Socio-Economic and Home Information

Jeff was adopted as an infant by a hearing impaired couple who were aware of his handicapping conditions. Both parents work as word processors for a computer company. The family lives in an older section of town in a renovated townhouse several blocks from the bus stop to work and near a small business area where they do most of their shopping. The family's social life centers around activities at the Deaf Center and "get-togethers" with deaf friends who serve as extended family. There appears to be no economic deprivation. Social services case workers periodically visit the family due to the nature of their handicapping conditions.

CURRENT MULTIDISCIPLINARY EVALUATION

This evaluation includes the following assessments: cognition, vision, hearing, speech/language, motor skills, and social development.

Psychological Evaluation

Previous Test Administered

Developmental Profile CA *3 years, 1 month* IQ *24*

Current Test Administered

The Callier-Azusa Scale (Cognition) CA *5 years, 1 month*
MA *1–4 months* IQ Range *Profoundly Mentally Retarded*

Testing Interpretation

Jeff was evaluated by interview with his teacher in his classroom. During the interview, Jeff laid on a bean bag. No attempt to move, vocalize, or interact with anyone was observed during this time. Teacher indicated that Jeff is very tactilely defensive and will pull away or turn away from caregivers when they attempt to interact with him. He inconsistently responds to extremely loud noises. Visually, Jeff will fixate on objects and appears to briefly look at a spot where a moving object was last seen. He appears to recognize his parents. He recognizes familiar objects and the beginning of a familiar activity. He tracks movements of people in the classroom. Jeff anticipates familiar events from whole body cues (e.g., opens mouth for food when placed in the usual feeding position). He will rock in response to an adult rocking him.

In summary, Jeff's skills fall below the 6 month level (estimate: 1–4 months level). Therefore, based on teacher report and observation, he appears to be functioning within the profoundly mentally handicapped range of intelligence.

School Psychologist

Vision Evaluation

Test Administered

Informal Optometrist Assessment

Testing Interpretation

Ophthalmological examination at age 3 years showed the eyes to be normal. No evidence of nystagmus, cataracts, or optic atrophy were outlined in the report and a 6 month follow-up was recommended.

At this screening, Jeff spontaneously fixated a penlight, flashlight, transilluminated lights and toys, and various brightly colored objects (e.g., pinwheel, red tip of gigglestick, reflective balloon, 3–4 inch diameter ball). Jeff fixated a penlight OD (right eye) and OS (left eye) up to 4–6 feet. OKN was elicited OD and OS up to the same distance. He did not visually attend the drum at a further distance. Fixations were central, steady, and maintained. Most of the time Jeff appeared binocular, however, at times he manifested a left exotropia. He could regain binocularity quickly and the near point of convergence was about 6 centimeters. Jeff made strong eye contact for 8–10 seconds. He visually tracked a clear plastic ball containing a rotating butterfly rolled on the floor horizontally before him and he followed the ball up to 6 feet away from himself.

External examination of the eye was not remarkable. The pupils were equal, round and reacted to light and accommodation. Jeff's visual functioning appears to be appropriate to his overall developmental level as determined by appropriate developmental assessment. His estimated corrected visual acuity may be better than 20/40 in the better eye.

In the classroom, Jeff directs his gaze to people as they approach him and will sometimes smile when approached by a familiar person. He tracks persons moving about the room using a whole head turn rather than following with his eyes alone. He attends and frequently seems interested in signs used by the caregiver. When tired or fussy, he will put his head down or try to fall asleep to avoid vision activities. Jeff does not reach for objects placed in his field of vision and he resists shaping of this activity, probably due to tactile defensiveness.

Optometrist

Hearing Evaluation

Test Administered

Behavioral Audiometry

Testing Interpretation

Jeff was seen for a routine hearing evaluation. Previous Brainstem Evoked Response Audiometry indicated a severe to profound predominantly sensorineural hearing loss, bilaterally. Jeff recently had myringotomies with tubes for treatment of middle ear problems. Jeff is presently utilizing binaural air conduction ear-level loaner hearing aids on trial basis. Jeff's aided and unaided auditory responses were assessed by observing behavioral responses to various auditory stimuli presented in a sound-field. No definite or repeatable responses were noted with or without the use of hearing aids. Results were as follows:

Stimulus	Aided/Unaided Hearing Level	Aided/Unaided Response
Monitored Live Voice	70dB/80dB	Possible Awareness/Startle
Squeaky Toy	90dB/90dB	Smile/Questionable
Happy Apple	80dB/90dB	Startle/No Response
Cricket Noisemaker	80dB/80dB	No Response/No Response
Bicycle Horn	80dB/85dB	Blink/No Response

Continued testing is recommended in order to more firmly establish the possible benefits Jeff receives from amplification.

Educational Audiologist

Communication Evaluation

Test Administered

Informal Speech/Language Pathologist Assessment

Testing Interpretation

Jeff functions communicatively at the 3–4 month level. Expressively, he cries or whines when frustrated or uncomfortable. He will sometimes smile when approached by a familiar person or during an activity he finds pleasurable. He usually does not vocalize when alone. Jeff will sometimes respond to speech stimulation from caregiver by making sounds or noises. His primary vocalizations are cries or whines to indicate displeasure for handling or a particular activity.

Receptively, Jeff shows an interest in signs by visually attending and responds correctly to signs such as "eat" and "drink." He is beginning to display an understanding of the sign for "up" by lifting his head and shoulders in anticipation of being picked up. As yet, he has not responded or attended to signs such as "stop" and "go" because he does not enjoy the activities connected with these signs and usually fusses throughout these work periods.

Speech/Language Pathologist

Motor Evaluation

Tests Administered

The Callier-Azusa Scale
Informal Physical Therapy Assessment

Testing Interpretation

Muscle Tone and Range of Motion. Jeff's muscle tone is generally floppy (hypotonia) underneath stiffness (hypertonia), probably caused by his active movement into stiff patterns, especially in trunk and legs, from his avoidance of touching. Touching and handling usually cause fussing and posturing into a position of retracted arms and stiff trunk and legs with feet tightly pointed up. Range of motion is passively within normal limits except for stiffness in his trunk.

Fine Motor Skills. Jeff functions at the 0–1 month level in fine motor skills. He holds his arms retracted and up, with hands fisted, avoiding bringing his hands to midline or batting, and he resists being manipulated in these skills. Tactile defensiveness has severely negatively impacted fine motor skills development.

Gross Motor Skills. Jeff appears to be functioning at the 4–5 month level in gross motor skills. He prefers lying on his back in his stiff position. He log rolls to either side onto his stomach. While on his stomach, he can lift his head but he will not prop on his forearms. He can move from one place to another with a wiggling movement. Head control is good in all positions and when moving from one position to another.

Jeff does not tolerate a standing position when using a prone stander. If he could tolerate handling without fussing and posturing into a stiff position, he would probably display better motor skills and better sitting balance, more purposeful upper extremity movement and protective extension in the arms.

Secondary Senses. Jeff experiences vestibular malfunctioning. When placed on a carpeted hanging swing, he fusses not only in response to the new texture, but to movement regardless how slight. Movements required for learning to sit, stand, and walk cause unpleasantness and perhaps nausea. Since accurate vestibular functioning is a prerequisite to balance and mobility, progress in mobility will be slight until his aversion to tactile stimuli is reduced and his toleration for proprioceptive-kinesthetic-vestibular stimulation increased.

Self-Help Skills: Feeding. Jeff appears to be functioning at the 6 month level in feeding skills. He does not need to have his table food ground if held at the sides of his mouth for chewing. Tongue thrust is much improved, no longer pushing food from the mouth. He still uses suckling to consume food in the middle of the mouth. Tactile defensiveness has decreased at the face to allow for jaw control as necessary. When drinking, he retracts his lips from the rim of the cup and does not assist in pulling liquid out of the cup. Therefore, liquid is lost while drinking.

Jeff can sometimes maintain an independent grasp on a spoon and assist in bringing it to his mouth, although he misses his mouth. He tolerates having his hand held on a cup.

Physical Therapist

Social Development

Test Administered

The Callier-Azusa Scale (Social Development) Level: *6–8 months*

Testing Interpretation

Jeff's social development was assessed by interviewing mother and his teachers. His overall social development appears to be at the 6–8 month level.

On *Interactions with Adults,* Jeff appears to be functioning at the 6–8 month level. He responds negatively to person-to-person contact as he is tactilely defensive. He studies or attends to adults by smiling, and appears to differentiate familiar and unfamiliar adults. He will play a game if the adult paces the game. He cries and fusses to gain an adult's attention and will attempt to maintain the interactions.

Jeff's *Interactions with the Environment* appear to be at the 6–8 month level. He shows awareness of the presence of light and tactile stimulation. He has a preferred eating schedule. He attempts to move or change positions and vocalizes to show discomfort. Jeff exhibits different vocalizations, expresses preferences for particular foods, differentiates between familiar and unfamiliar environments, anticipates familiar events from cues.

Jeff's *Interactions with Other Children* appear to be at the 6 month level. He shows awareness of the presence of other children and smiles or vocalizes to other children's faces.

Educational Diagnostician

Evaluation Summary

Jeff is a 5 year, 4 months old student attending the Preschool Program for Severely Handicapped Students. Current psychological evaluation indicates that Jeff is functioning within the profoundly mentally handicapped range of intelligence with a mental age of less than six months. During the interview with his teacher he made no attempt to move, vocalize, or interact with anyone. He does not manipulate objects, but visually inspects them and appears to continue to look at a spot where a moving object was last seen.

Visually, Jeff spontaneously fixated various lights and toys and brightly colored objects up to 4–6 feet. Fixations were central, steady, and maintained. Most of the time he appeared binocular. Jeff visually tracked toys horizontally. His visual functioning appears to be appropriate to his overall developmental level. Jeff's estimated visual acuity may be 20/40 in the better eye.

Previous BES Audiometry indicated a severe to profound sensorineural hearing loss bilaterally. He recently had myringotomies with tubes for treatment of middle ear problems. Jeff was unresponsive to auditory stimuli with or without the use of amplification. Possible aided auditory responses including eye blink, startle, cessation of activity, or smile have been noted to noisemakers or monitored live voice at levels of 60dB HL to 90dB HL. Minimal benefits have been seen from amplification.

In the classroom Jeff cries or whines when frustrated or uncomfortable. He will sometimes smile when approached by a familiar person or during an activity he finds pleasurable. He responds to signs "eat" and "drink" and is beginning to understand "up." He does not vocalize in response to others, but does emit a vocalization "his sound."

Developmentally, Jeff appears to be functioning at the following levels:

Developmental Skills	*Functioning Level*
Cognition	1–4 months
Communication	3–4 months
Fine Motor	0–1 months
Gross Motor	4–5 months
Feeding	6 months
Social	6–8 months

Jeff has a medical diagnosis of cerebral palsy.

Case Manager

DIAGNOSIS: Severely/Multihandicapped (hearing impaired, profound mental retardation, physical impairment)

RE-EVALUATION REPORT
HEATHER

Age: 11 years, 11 months
Grade: Ungraded Intermediate Class for Severely Handicapped
Date: April , 19___

Background and Educational Concerns

Reason for Referral

Heather is an 11 year, 11 month old student attending an ungraded intermediate-age class for severely handicapped students. She has attended various classes for severely handicapped students since age 3 years when she was originally diagnosed at school as being severely handicapped. This is a special request evaluation regarding placement needs due to Heather's increase in inappropriate behaviors and female maturational concerns.

Health

School health records indicate that Heather has no outstanding medical concerns. Immunizations are current. She is ambulatory, but needs a ramp.

Medical records indicate a history of motor and mental retardation with secondary blindness. At age 3 years, Heather had corrective eye surgery for frequent crossed eyes.

Visual History

On initial evaluation at age 3 years Heather exhibited the following visual behaviors: attended to and reached out for light and objects placed in a horizontal plane at a distance of 12 inches or closer, did not appear to discriminate visually, no tracking of light or objects. At age 7 years, the End-of-Year Report indicated that Heather inconsistently turned her head toward a penlight, reached out for a cup after turning her head toward it, and showed no evidence of tracking or eye contact.

The End-of-Year Report at age 9 years indicated that Heather appears to have better peripheral vision than central vision. She can reach out for a small food stimulus on the right and left, upper and lower visual planes. She does not reach for a food stimulus centrally unless presented to the side first, then moved in to a distance of about 8 inches from the face.

Auditory History

During Heather's initial school evaluation at age 3 years, she responded consistently to musical toys, but inconsistently responded to verbal language. At age 7 years, Heather showed an awareness to sound at 30dB to 40dB HL, and appeared to localize to sound. Audiological testing at age 9 years indicated hearing adequate for reception of speech and language. Heather responded by cessation of self-stimulation. She localized at levels of 30dB to 40dB HL to noisemakers and live voice. She smiled to praise, "Good girl, Heather." In the classroom she smiles to voice and music, and at times will cease self-stimulation when directed. Audiological testing at age 10 years revealed normal hearing for at least one ear. Heather responded to sounds at 20dB HL.

Developmental History

Heather's previous evaluations indicate development as follows:

Developmental Skills	*At 2 yrs. 10 mo.*	*At 7 yrs. 9 mo.*	*At 9 yrs. 10 mo.*
Cognition	1–2 months	4–6 months	12 months
Receptive Language	0–2 months	9–12 months	12–14 months
Expressive Language	0–1 months	6 months	6–10 months
Fine Motor	4–6 months	8–9 months	8–9 months
Gross Motor	7–8 months	8–9 months	9–10 months
Self-Help	0–2 months	8–9 months	12 months

Socio-Economic and Home Information

Heather is the youngest of three children; Jeff and Kate are in high school. Father teaches social studies at the Middle School. Mother is a real estate agent who specializes in selling apartment buildings. English is the language of the home. The family lives in an average middle-class settled neighborhood in a well-kept brick home. Both parents, also, work during the summer due to the high costs of Heather's care.

Currently, parents are considering an alternative placement because they are experiencing significant difficulty controlling Heather's inappropriate behaviors and female maturation concerns at home. There appears to be no socio-economic deprivation.

CURRENT MULTIDISCIPLINARY EVALUATION

This re-evaluation includes the following assessments: cognition, vision, hearing, communication, physical, social, and behavioral skills.

Psychological Evaluation

Test Administered

The Callier-Azusa Scale (Cognitive)

CA *11 years, 9 months* MA *Below 18 months* IQ *Profound*

Testing Interpretation

Heather is an average-sized 11 year, 11 month old girl. She was observed as she finished lunch in her classroom. Her teacher and the teacher assistant were interviewed for this report.

Heather engages in numerous self-stimulatory behaviors including hand flapping and biting, head shaking, smacking sounds, tongue clicking, rocking in chair, rubbing hands and breasts. Behavioral concerns include biting others and throwing things when angry, and emitting "primal screams" for no apparent reason.

Heather can ambulate independently short distances in the classroom, but requires arm support and/or nudging in the hallway. Last year's hearing test was within normal range; this year stimulatory behaviors interfered with testing. Central vision remains questionable, but Heather is able to use peripheral vision when she chooses to attend. She can feed herself with her fingers, with a spoon is emerging. She drinks from a mug independently. Toileting at school is a goal.

Current evaluation indicates mastery of some skills up to the 18 months level. At the 1–4 months level, Heather systematically repeats movements in which the focus is on the stimulation of the body. She anticipates familiar events from whole body cues (e.g., opens mouth for food when in the usual feeding position). She responds to cues from another person by participating in modification of her movement. She uses at least one behavior in exploring an object and uses consistent schemas in interacting with a new toy or object. Visually, Heather recognizes a familiar object or beginning of a familiar activity. Inconsistently, she demonstrates a visually-directed reach and grasp. Heather moves her head to locate the source of sound (moves to right or left only). She makes spontaneous vocalizations without distress and shows a positive response to familiar sounds or movements by smiling or laughing. She sometimes mouths objects placed in her hands.

At the 5–7 months level, Heather demonstrates visually-directed reaching in bringing her closed hand up to an object and shapes her hand in anticipation of securing an object. She will drop one or both objects held in hands to obtain a third. She performs consistent actions in response to familiar gestures (e.g., patting table, shaking toy). Heather has integrated simple schemas such as banging objects on a table and uses simple motor schemas independent of a table surface. She drops or throws objects.

At the 8–12 month level, Heather sometimes can secure a hidden object. She inconsistently combines typical behaviors to intentionally obtain an object or achieve a goal. Sometimes she anticipates a routine event from environmental cues. Sometimes she pushes an obstruction out of the way to obtain a desired object. She uses some form of locomotion as a means to obtain an out of reach object. If an object is placed on or between supports, she will not move the support but goes directly for the object.

At the 13–18 months level, Heather recognizes that other people can obtain an object or perform a task for her. She localizes the source of sound by turning her head directly toward the source. Heather can give the sign for "eat" when she wants more food.

Heather's skills are splintered up to the 18 months level. Poor attending interferes with skill development. She has not established object permanence but will search the pocket of her bib for extra food after eating so this may be emerging. Food is the only successful motivator used to control her inappropriate behaviors. She will use the signs "eat," "drink," and "potty."

In summary, Heather is functioning within a profoundly mentally handicapped range of intelligence. Self-stimulatory behaviors severely impede her ability to attend to her environment and, thus, develop new skills. A diagnosis of behavior disordered should be considered along with the diagnosis of mentally handicapped.

School Psychologist

Vision Evaluation
(Optometric Screening)

Ocular history, ophthalmological, and neurological diagnoses from age 2 years and 4 years indicated vision impairment due to general neurologic deficiency. It was felt that Heather had light perception and perhaps form perception. Fundus examination was normal at that time. Heather had eye muscle surgery at age 3 years, 2 months.

At this evaluation, Heather positioned her eyes in extreme right gaze using a head turn to the left to facilitate this right gaze throughout most of the examination. She seemed to demonstrate an awareness to a penlight and transilluminated penlight (red) by quieting all her movements and getting her head positioned as described above. This response was repeatable. No "direct" fixational response was ever made in contrast to the "eccentric" (off center") type gaze. Visual fields cannot be quantified, however, certain foodstuffs of 10 mm. in size or larger when brought from periphery to central about 8–10 inches from Heather's eyes, seem to pass through areas of field that alerted Heather to the location of the food. She demonstrated amazing eye-hand accuracy using the eccentric gaze.

Heather did not demonstrate the ability to track, nor did she make direct eye contact. Eye movements did appear conjugate. Occasional nystagmoid eye movements were noted. Because of the lack of direct fixational response and the use of eccentric gaze, central visual acuity may be estimated as 20/200 or less in the better eye. Based on the possible loss or non-use of central visual acuity (etiology unknown), Heather could be considered to meet the definition of legal blindness.

Optometrist

Hearing Evaluation

Tests Administered

Impedance Test
Behavioral Audiometry

Testing Interpretation

Heather was seen for routine hearing evaluation. Impedance test for middle ear function could not be obtained due to Heather's uncooperative behavior. Her hearing was assessed by observing behavioral responses to various auditory stimuli presented in a sound-field. Results are as follows:

Stimulus	*Hearing Level*	*Response*
Monitored Live Voice	20dB	Smile
Drum	20dB	Smile
Squeaky Toy	20dB	Smile
Raggedy Ann Rattle	20dB	Cessation/Smile
Happy Apple	20dB	Cessation/Smile
Cricket Noisemaker	20dB	Localization
Bicycle Horn	20dB	Localization

Overall test results indicate normal hearing for at least one ear. Heather has been seen at school for 10 previous hearing evaluations which all indicated normal hearing for at least one ear.

Educational Audiologist

Communication Evaluation (Informal Assessment)

Receptively, Heather appears to be functioning at the 12–18 months developmental level. She responds correctly to simple commands such as "stand up," "sit," "scoop," "come," and "stop," about 10% of the time. Heather signs "eat" and "drink" correctly about 90% of the time at mealtime or when expecting an edible reward. She frequently responds to "no" when paired with appropriate gesture and tone.

Expressively, Heather is functioning on the 6–12 months developmental level. She verbalizes /ee/, /et/, and /ma-ma/.

Classroom Teacher

Motor Evaluation

Test Administered

The Callier-Azusa Scale

Testing Interpretation

Gross Motor. Gross motor skills are at the 12 months level. Heather can walk on flat, smooth ground independently for short distances. She walks indefinitely with verbal/tactile cues to direct her. She will take as much support as offered by caregivers. Heather walks around large objects, but will trip over low-lying ones. She is able to get up and down from the floor with arm rotation, help and encouragement. Heather's main motor schema is prone or side lying and rocking. She is able to descend and ascend steps holding on with one hand on the rail and one hand held by caregiver. Stair walking is not independent due to inconsistent foot placement.

Fine Motor. Fine motor skills appear to be at the 6–12 months developmental level. Heather has individualization of fingers in self-stimulatory motions. Pressure on objects is decreased. Heather picks up blocks with a palmar grasp, and smaller objects with thumb against the side of the index finger with wrist downward. She does not play appropriately with toys. She picks up finger foods with her right hand using a later pincer grasp.

Self-Help Skills: Feeding. Heather has very definite food preferences. She uses a built-up spoon with a weak right-hand grasp. She seeks out and picks up finger foods with her right hand using a lateral pincer grasp. Heather signs "eat" and reaches for a person when she wants help. She drinks from a cup or straw. Heather has appropriate chewing and tongue lateralization. She does not bite off a piece of sandwich appropriately. Scooping has improved over the past year, but a completely independent scooping pattern is not present. Feeding skills are at the 16 months level.

Self-Help Skills: Toileting. Heather is not toilet scheduled. She averages between 6–10 accidents per week. Additionally, Heather has begun menstruation.

Self-Help Skills: Dressing. When an arm of a jacket is partially removed, Heather will take off the rest of the arm of the jacket. She requires hand-over-hand in pulling or pushing down pants. Dressing skills are at the 16 months level.

Physical Therapist

Social Evaluation

Test Administered

The Callier-Azusa Scale (Social Development) Level: *5-6 months*

Testing Interpretation

Heather's *Interactions with Adults* appear to be at the 5–6 months level. She shows awareness of the presence of an adult by turning her head to scan the person and then she smiles. Heather sometimes appears to visually scan adults using peripheral vision. She attends to caregivers when they call her name. She responds to an adult's attempt to interact by smiling. She interacts with adults using eat/drink sign to let her needs be known.

Heather's *Interactions with the Environment* appear to be at the six month level. She shows awareness of the presence of light, sound, and tactile stimulation. She shows a preferred eating schedule and exhibits food preferences. She moves and changes her position. Heather exhibits self-stimulatory behaviors. She vocalizes to show discomfort when hungry, wet, or in pain. Heather responds to being kissed. She is aware of body parts and uses them for self-stimulation. She differentiates familiar and unfamiliar environments. Heather reacts to frustrating situations by tantrum behaviors. She anticipates a familiar event in the presence of several cues.

Heather's *Interactions with Other Children* appear to be at the 0–1 month level. She shows awareness of the presence of another child especially if they are crying. She does not respond to or interact with other children.

Educational Diagnostician: Respondent: Mother

Behavior Evaluation
(Informal Assessment)

Self-stimulation of numerous types continue. When demands are made on Heather, she may bite her hands and try to bite others or throw objects. Periodically, for unknown reasons and on an indeterminate schedule, Heather emits loud, high pitched "primal screams," which frighten the other students. She avoids doing tasks by engaging in self-stimulation or when physically assisted to respond, she will go completely limp and slumps to the floor.

A number of techniques have been attempted to intervene with Heather's self-stimulating behaviors. Often, however, when one set of behaviors is briefly stopped, she engages in another set of self-stimulatory behaviors. These behaviors interfere with all learning activities.

Classroom Teacher

Evaluation Summary

Heather is an 11 year, 11 months old student attending an ungraded intermediate program for severely handicapped students. Current psychological evaluation indicates functioning within a profoundly mentally handicapped range of intelligence with a mental age of below 18 months.

Visual evaluation indicates that Heather did not track, made no direct eye contact, and exhibited no fixational response. Heather positioned her eyes in extreme right gaze using a head turn to the left to facilitate the right gaze. Using this gaze, she could locate foodstuffs of 10 mm. in size and about 8–10 inches from her eyes. Central acuity may be estimated as 20/200 or less in the better eye. Heather appears to be legally blind.

Hearing evaluation indicated responses to speech and noisemakers at 20dB HL in a sound-field. Heather's hearing appears normal for at least one ear. Auditory responses appear commensurate with her overall development.

Heather's developmental skills are as follows:

Developmental Skills	*Levels*
Cognition	Below 18 months
Receptive Language	12–18 months
Expressive Language	6–12 months
Gross Motor	12 months
Fine Motor	6–12 months
Feeding	16 months
Dressing	16 months
Social Development	5–6 months

Inappropriate behavior is a significant concern. Heather responds to commands only about 10% of the time. Self-stimulatory behaviors of numerous types continue. When demands are made on Heather she bites her hands and tries to bite others, she throws things, or goes limp and slumps to the floor. The school psychologist recommended consideration of a diagnosis of behavior disordered due to the many self-stimulatory behaviors interfering with the learning. Self-stimulatory behaviors interfered with testing, and impede her ability to attend to her environment and develop new skills. Aggressive behaviors toward teachers and others is a significant concern because of her adult size.

Additional concerns that the intermediate grade classroom for severely multihandicapped students functioning at preschool levels is not appropriately equipped to handle include feminine sanitary needs during menstruation.

Case Manager

DIAGNOSIS: Severely/Multihandicapped (vision impaired, profoundly mentally retarded, behavior disordered)

RE-EVALUATION REPORT
RANDY

Age: 15 years, 3 months
Grade: Ungraded Adolescent Program for Severely Handicapped
Date: April , 19___

Background and Educational Concerns

Reason for Referral

Randy is a 15 year, 3 months old student attending an ungraded adolescent program for severely multihandicapped students. Randy has attended various programs at this Special Day School since he was 3 years, 3 months old, when he was initially diagnosed as severely multihandicapped. This is a routine 3 year re-evaluation.

Health

School health records indicate immunizations are current. Randy takes tegritol and phenobarbitol at home for a seizure disorder. He takes no medication at school. He has flat feet but no treatment is recommended at this time. Randy is ambulatory but he needs a ramp with railing.

Medical records indicate a history of the following concerns: pneumococcal meningitis complicated by motor seizure activity and respiratory arrest, hydrocephalus (shunted at age 5 months), seizure disorder, hemiparesis, possible deafness and blindness.

Vision History

On initial evaluation at age 3 years, 3 months, Randy demonstrated the presence of right peripheral vision, but the presence of central vision was undetermined. The Progress Report at age 5 years stated that Randy gave brief eye contact when commanded. At age 8 years the Progress Report indicated that Randy used his right visual field more than left, turned to see a light source, turned his head to see an object rather than moving his eyes, tracked vertically and horizontally, used a visually directed reach and grasp.

The End-of-Year Report at age 10 years stated that Randy avoided eye contact to avoid work, fixated on objects, possessed a visually directed reach and grasp, and could see in all planes but preferred horizontal.

The Report indicated that Randy's vision is functional for all purposes including feeding, fine motor, and locomotion.

Hearing History

Auditory evaluation at age 3 years, 3 months indicated that Randy inconsistently startled to loud noises and responded to soft sounds close to his ear by smiling and vocalizing. By age 6 years, audiological testing indicated auditory development at the 7–9 months level with localization to noisemakers at 20dB HL. Hearing testing at ages 7 and 8 years reported normal tympanograms for both ears, acoustic reflexes elicited within normal limits, normal hearing sensitivity, and peripheral hearing mechanism adequate for the reception of speech and language. Hearing testing at age 10 years indicated responses to live voice at 15dB, normal tympanograms for both ears, and essentially normal hearing. In the classroom, Randy responds to simple commands at conversational speech levels, enjoys playing rhythm band instruments, and claps hands and taps feet to music.

Developmental History

A picture of Randy's learning rate can be derived from examination of his progress in developmental skills at various ages as follows:

Developmental Skills	*At 3 years*	*At 5 years*	*At 7 years*	*At 12 years*
Cognition	0–1 mo.	1–4 mo.	6–7 mo.	8–12 mo.
Receptive Language	0–1 mo.	3–4 mo.	6 mo.	16–18 mo.
Expressive Language	3–4 mo.	3–4 mo.	6 mo.	16–18 mo.
Gross Motor	10–11 mo.	11–12 mo.	13 mo.	18–24 mo.
Fine Motor	6–7 mo.	9 mo.	10–11 mo.	12–14 mo.
Socialization			5 mo.	7–8 mo.
Feeding				24 mo.
Dressing				12 mo.

Socio-Economic and Home Information

English is the language of the home. Randy's father works for the State as a supervisor on a road construction crew and mother is a homemaker. His two older brothers and older sister are married and have young children. The family lives in a small community and the parents own their older comfortable home. Parents are concerned about Randy's living circumstances as they near retirement age. They are considering placement in the group home newly constructed in a small town about 13 miles away. The school social worker makes periodic visits to the home to assist parents in dealing with problems and concerns. There is no economic deprivation.

CURRENT MULTIDISCIPLINARY EVALUATION

This evaluation includes the following assessments: cognition, vision, hearing, motor, social, behavior, developmental, and prevocational skills.

Psychological Evaluation

Previous Tests Administered

Battelle Developmental Inventory CA *7 years, 6 months* MA *6-7 months*

Current Test Administered

Cattell Infant Intelligence Scale

CA *15 years, 2 months* MA *9.6 months* IQ *Profound*

Testing Interpretation

Randy was evaluated in his classroom while seated at a small table. Both hearing and vision are present. Randy has splinter skills up to the 12 months level. Communication skills mastered at the 1–4 months level include making spontaneous vocalizations without distress; showing a positive response to familiar sounds or movements by smiling or laughing; vocalizing in response to vocalizations produced by others, cooing, babbling; imitating cooing sounds. At the 5–7 months level, Randy makes an effort to deliberately imitate known sounds and movements.

Visually, at the 1–4 months level, Randy continues to look at a spot where a moving object was last seen, shifts gaze from one stimulus to another, tracks a slow moving object in a 180° horizontal arc, demonstrates visually directed reach and grasp, visually inspects objects placed in his hands. At the 5–7 months level, he rotates objects in his hands and visually inspects all sides. At the 8–12 months level, he realizes that an object continues to exist after he can no longer see it and differentiates sizes of objects.

At the 8–12 months level, Randy's visual-motor skills include the following: combines two typical behaviors to intentionally obtain an object or achieve a goal, pushes an obstruction out of the way to obtain a desired object, pulls a support to obtain an object placed on it, uses locomotion as a means to obtain an out-of-reach object, reaches directly above to get an object.

Auditorially, at the 13–18 months level, Randy localizes the source of sound by turning his head directly toward the source. He anticipates a routine event from environmental cues.

In summary, Randy is performing within the profoundly retarded range with a mental age of 9.6 months with splinter skills to 12 months.

School Psychologist

Vision Evaluation

Tests Administered

Informal Optometric Assessment
The Callier-Azusa Scale (Vision and Visual-Motor Subscales)

Testing Interpretation

Medical information outlined at the time Randy was an infant indicated poor fixational ability and an impression of cortical blindness. Examination of the eye revealed the fundus to be within normal limits. No recent information documenting Randy's ocular health or vision status was available.

At this evaluation, Randy spontaneously fixated a penlight, flashlight, transilluminated objects, foodstuffs, and toys with the O.D. (right eye) and O.S. (left eye). He manifested a large angle alternating exotropia. Today he seemed to prefer the O.S., however, his teachers feel they observe him to use O.D. Fixations were central, steady, and maintained for 3–4 seconds, again the O.S. seemed slightly stronger at this time.

Randy made strong eye contact up to 5–8 seconds. He tracked foodstuffs and a small pendant on a necklace horizontally and vertically, and crossed the midline with each eye. OKN was elicited up to 3–4 feet with O.D. and O.S. Randy reached for a pendant (4–5 mm) at 18 inches with fair eye-hand accuracy. He also reached for small foodstuffs up to 24 inches.

Confrontation testing with a finger, food item of interest, or even with a larger object (cup) indicated there might be left visual field restriction.

Randy resisted occlusion to test each eye individually, so the suspected loss may be O.D. (right), O.S. (left), or O.U. (both). He consistently did not respond visually to the items listed previously when they were moved in from his upper left, left, and lower left visual fields almost to the midline. Randy did respond visually by fixation when they were visually picked up in the right visual field. Even though Randy was distracted by occlusion, I suspect the field loss may be some degree of a homongnous hemanopsia as the response was similar whether he fixed with the O.D. or O.S. There also has been a history of a possible left field defect.

Visual acuity cannot be definitively measured and Randy does not use his vision appropriate to the overall developmental level. "Visual-motor" and "Visual" subscales of *The Callier-Azusa Scale* indicated vision function at 5 months and 8 months levels respectively. Part of the functional non-use of vision may be related back to an actual visual field loss.

Optometrist

Hearing Evaluation

Tests Administered

Impedance Test
Behavioral Audiometry

Testing Interpretation

Results of Randy's last five hearing evaluations at school have indicated that hearing is adequate for the reception of speech and language or essentially normal hearing for at least one ear.

Randy was seen for a routine hearing evaluation. His hearing was assessed by observing behavioral responses to various auditory stimuli presented in a sound-field. Results were as follows:

Stimulus	*Hearing Level*	*Response*
Monitored Live Voice	10dB	Localization
Drum	20dB	Cessation
Squeaky Toy	15dB	Laugh
Raggedy Ann Rattle	20dB	Laugh
Happy Apple	20dB	Cessation
Cricket Noisemaker	30dB	Localization

Impedance test for middle ear function shows normal tympanograms for both ears. Results indicate essentially normal hearing for at least one ear.

Educational Audiologist

Communication Evaluation (Informal Assessment)

Receptively, Randy responds to simple commands in normal conversational tones with fair consistency. He stops on-going action when told "No" accompanied by appropriate gesture and tone. Randy responds appropriately to the following directives: Stop, Randy; Stand Up; Eat. When told "Time to go potty," Randy will walk toward the bathroom.

Expressively, Randy approximates "good" when pleased, clapping his hands. He signs "drink" regularly, and "food" when interested. Randy smiles, laughs, hugs, and pouts appropriately. He appears to be functioning communicatively at the 16–18 months level.

Speech/Language Pathologist

Motor Evaluation (Informal Assessment)

Gross Motor Skills. Randy's muscle tone is hypertonic in left extremities. He has a limitation in range of motion with left overhead shoulder flexion and left elbow extension. His hip flexor tightens bilaterally. Randy's motor skills are greatly dependent on his degree of motivation or the dosage level of his medication. He is able to ambulate independently, requiring standby assistance due to possible seizures. Randy tends to lean heavily on the caretaker if available to him. He ambulates with a crouched, shuffling, flat foot gait. He is able to get up from a chair and to seat himself in a chair. He crawls, tall and half kneels, and pulls himself to stand along a supported surface. He ascends and descends stairs leaning on the railing. Most of his movements are sluggish, often unsteady. Upper extremity protective responses are present forwards and sideways. It should be noted that Randy's energy level is considerably increased over the past year. Gross motor skills appear to be at the 12–18 months developmental level.

Fine Motor Skills. Randy relies on his right hand for functional activities. Primary fine motor schemas include mouthing, banging, and shaking objects. He puts objects in and takes them out of containers, but shows no interest in sorting objects. Fine motor skills appear to be at the 12–14 months level.

Self-Help Skills: Feeding. Randy has good oral skills with tongue lateralization, chewing, and normal swallowing responses. He has improved scooping with a regular spoon and high sided dish and he continues to work on using a fork with 10% accuracy in poking. He drinks independently using glasses or cups without handles, and inconsistently puts them down on the table after drinking without spillage. Feeding skills appear to be at the 24 months level.

Self-Help Skills: Dressing. Randy is much improved in removing his jacket when one arm is started for him, and is starting to remove "one and a half" arms. He will usually remove an overhead shirt when one arm is partially removed. He does not pull a shirt on overhead—removes it instead. Dressing skills appear to be at the 12 months developmental level.

Self-Help Skills: Toileting. Randy regularly makes bowel movements in the toilet and has apparently overcome an apparent fear of the toilet enough that he urinates several times a week after a bowel movement. However, he still prefers to hold—often urinating in his pants right after getting off the toilet. He appears to be functioning at the 12 months level in toileting skills.

Physical Therapist

Home Social Behavior

Test Administered

The Callier-Azusa Scale (Social Development) Level: *10–12 months*

Testing Interpretation

Randy's *Interactions with Adults* appear to be at the 12 months level. He shows awareness of the presence of an adult; responds to person-to-person contact; sometimes attends to an adult visually, auditorially, or tactilely; responds with at least a single behavior to an adult's attempt to interact. Randy initiates an interaction by pulling on an adult to get their attention. He claps his hands when he wakes up to gain attention. He attempts to maintain contact with familiar adults and sometimes seeks to sustain interactions. He responds to simple commands.

His *Interactions with the Environment* appear to be at the 10–12 months level. Randy shows awareness of light, sound, or tactile stimulation. He shows a preferred eating pattern and expresses definite preferences for food. He changes positions and exhibits self-stimulatory behaviors. Randy responds to tactile stimulation, exhibits different vocalizations, and shows an awareness of body movements and body parts. He differentiates familiar and unfamiliar environments, but does not respond to noticeable changes in familiar environments. He reacts to frustrating situations with tantrums, self-stimulation, or withdrawal.

Randy's *Interactions with Other Children* appear to be at the 12 months level. He shows awareness of the presence of another child, responds to another child's presence, smiles or vocalizes to other children, explores another child as an object. Randy attempts to initiate interactions with other children and responds to another child's attempt to interact.

Educational Diagnostician; Respondent: Mother

Behavior Evaluation

Test Administered

AAMD Adaptive Behavior Scale, School Edition Level: *Below TMR*

Testing Interpretation

Randy's overall performance indicates that his behavior is significantly lower than that of a Trainable Mentally Retarded student.

Personal Self-Sufficiency. In terms of independent functioning, Randy is almost totally dependent on others. Randy's strengths include the following skills: feeding himself with a spoon, sitting without support, lifts cup or glass, grasps with thumb and finger, has effective use of right arm. He is totally dependent on others for toileting, personal cleanliness, dressing, etc.

Community Self-Sufficiency. Randy's performance reflected severe deficit functioning in the area of community self-sufficiency. He is somewhat ambulatory (walking with head hanging down, feet apart, dragging or shuffling feet), and can go around the class room alone, but not the school. In terms of language development, Randy does not speak. He communicates by nodding his head or smiling to express happiness; pointing, signing, or making vocal noises to indicate wants; chuckling or laughing when happy; making vocal noises to express anger.

Personal-Social Responsibility. Randy's behavior in this area appears to be in the severe deficit range compared to a trainable mentally retarded (TMR) child of the same age. His strength in the area of attention includes being able to pay attention to a purposeful activity for at least five minutes. Randy's behavior primarily reflects withdrawn and inactive behavior in the following ways: frequent sitting or standing in one position for a long period of time, frequent falling asleep in a chair, occasionally lying on the floor all day not seeming to react to anything and not being aware of surroundings, apathetic and unresponsive, demonstrating a blank fixed stare/expression.

Social Adjustment. In the area of social adjustment, Randy's behavior appears similar to that of a TMR child of the same age. Randy demonstrates the following unacceptable oral habits: audibly grinds teeth, chews or sucks fingers, chews or sucks clothing or other inedibles, and puts everything into his mouth. He does not exhibit strange and unacceptable habits and does not remove or tear off his clothing. He is afraid to climb or descend stairs. Randy constantly fidgets with his hands.

Personal Adjustment. Randy's personal adjustment represents an area of severe deficit as compared to a trainable mentally handicapped child. He frequently engages in the following stereotyped behaviors: hands constantly in motion; slaps, scratches, or rubs self continuously; waves or shakes parts of the body continually; moves or rolls head back and forth; rocks body back and forth. Randy frequently demonstrates the following inappropriate interpersonal manners: blows on others' faces, kisses or licks others, hugs or squeezes others, hangs onto others and does not let go. Randy's disturbing vocal or speech habits include making growling, humming, or other noises.

Summary. Randy's behavior represents a significant deficient deviation not only from average students and educable mentally retarded students, but also from trainable mentally retarded students. Randy's functioning reflects almost total dependence on others for life support activities.

Educational Diagnostician

Social Worker Report

On September 18, 19___, Randy's teachers and therapists approached me re: Randy's increased seizure activity. At one point, he had fallen and hit his head, so there was a concern that he may need to wear a helmet for head protection. I consulted with his mother and she agreed that we could try a helmet with him here at school. There was a concern that he might not tolerate it. Randy's mother also told me that his seizure medication had not been changed in over one year, but he had recently been checked by his physician. Randy had been seizure-free for almost six months, but they began again shortly before school started this fall.

At the IEP conference, I told Randy's mother that he tolerated the helmet well here, and that he only wears it for walking. I suggested where she might purchase one if she chooses (it is a hockey-type helmet). We also discussed the possibility that I would train the family in how to follow the toileting program begun at school, as soon as he has shows consistency.

School Social Worker

Prevocational Evaluation

Randy is a severely multihandicapped adolescent functioning within the sensorimotor stage at 10–18 months developmental level in all areas. At this time, he is not an appropriate candidate for sheltered-workshop placement because of the following: (1) lack of personal self-sufficiency in terms of toileting, personal cleanliness, and dressing; (2) limited communication skills both receptive and expressive; (3) lack of motivation and interest in performing simple prevocational tasks; (4) unacceptable oral habits; (5) stereotyped behaviors and inappropriate interpersonal manners; and (6) disturbing vocal habits. Randy does not possess any of the Competitive Employment Survival Skills.

Prevocational Teacher

Evaluation Summary

Randy is a 15 year, 3 months old severely multihandicapped student. Current cognitive evaluation indicates that he is functioning within the profoundly retarded range with a mental age of 9.6 months.

Visually, Randy spontaneously fixated lights, foodstuffs, and toys with the right and left eye; and tracked horizontally and vertically with each eye. Fixations were central, steady, and maintained for 3–4 seconds. He made strong eye contact up to 5–8 seconds. Confrontation testing indicated there might be left visual field restriction. Visual-motor skills appear to be at the 5 months level and visual skills at the 8 months level. Thus, Randy does not use his vision appropriate to his overall developmental level.

Randy has essentially normal hearing for at least one ear. At this evaluation, he responded to speech and noisemakers from 10dB to 30dB HL. Randy's observed behavioral responses appear commensurate with his overall developmental level.

Randy's developmental skills indicate a slow rate of progress as follows:

Developmental Skill	*Functioning Level*
Cognition	9–12 months
Fine Motor	12–14 months
Gross Motor	12–18 months
Language	16–18 months
Feeding	24 months
Dressing & Toileting	12 months
Social Behavior	10–12 months

Randy's adaptive behavior represents a significant deficit from the behavior of average, EMR, and TMR students. He appears to be functioning within the severely handicapped range in personal self-sufficiency, community self-sufficiency, personal-social responsibility, and personal adjustment. In the area of social adjustment, Randy is functioning similarly to a TMR student of the same age. He has unacceptable oral habits, stereotyped behaviors, inappropriate interpersonal manners, and disturbing vocal habits.

He has a medical diagnosis of hemiparesis. His muscle tone is hypertonic in left extremities. He takes medication for a seizure disorder.

Case Manager

DIAGNOSIS: Severely Multihandicapped (vision impaired, profoundly mentally retarded, physically impaired, other health impaired)

Chapter Five

CASES OF BEHAVIOR DISORDERED STUDENTS

Disturbed behaviors are frequently categorized as mild-moderate behavior disorders (aggressive behaviors, withdrawn behaviors) and severe-profound behavior disorders. Mild-moderate behavior disordered children (IQs around 90) are usually educated in the public school systems in self-contained classrooms, gradually mainstreamed to the regular classroom as they learn to control their inappropriate behaviors. Severe-profound behavior disordered students are frequently educated in special day schools or hospitals. Many severe-profound behavior disordered children and youth are untestable; those who are testable generally function as severely retarded individuals.

Preschool Age/Grade: Regina
Primary Age/Grade: Craig
Intermediate Age/Grade: Gary
  See Also: Heather
Secondary Age/Grade: Daniel

EVALUATION REPORT
REGINA

Age: 5 years, 4 months
Grade: Kindergarten
Date: October , 19___

Background and Educational Concerns

Reason for Referral

Regina is a 5 year, 4 months old kindergarten student attending Oakwood Elementary School. Her family moved here from out-of-state just before school started. There is no previous academic or pre-kindergarten testing results.

Regina has been referred by her kindergarten teacher due to her inappropriate and immature behaviors. She appears to have no impulse control. She is aggressive: bites, hits, kicks, and pushes other children. If someone has a toy that she decides she wants, she tackles them and fights until they give her the toy. She never follows directions, cannot seem to sit still, and does no school work. Nothing the teacher has tried works. A teacher aide takes Regina out of the classroom at regularly scheduled times to reduce disruption and tries to work with her individually.

Health

Immunizations are current. A school physical examination just prior to beginning school indicated no specific problems.

Vision and Hearing Screenings: Normal Range Acuities

Speech and Language Screenings

Speech and language screenings indicate functioning at the 4 year level. Speech and language evaluations are recommended.

Socio-Economic and Home Information

English is the language of the home. Regina is the youngest of five children and the only one at home, the other children being significantly older. Several of her older brothers and sisters have children her age. Father is a butcher at a local market and mother is a word processor for a small business company.

Regina has been "very forward" since she was quite young. Mother indicates that preschool years were a constant search for a new day care center or babysitter because of Regina's behavior. She is "very different" from the other children when they were her age, and "very different" from the grandchildren. Regina refuses to mind. Parents have no idea how to control Regina as neither spankings for bad behavior nor rewards for good behavior have consistently worked.

CURRENT MULTIDISCIPLINARY EVALUATION

This evaluation includes the following assessments: intelligence, perception, communication, motor, preacademics, behavior, and social skills.

Psychological Evaluation

Tests Administered

Wechsler Preschool and Primary Scale of Intelligence (WPPSI)

Verbal IQ	*69*	Performance IQ	*79*	Full Scale IQ	*70*
Information	*6*	Animal House	*7*		
Vocabulary	*5*	Picture Completion	*6*		
Arithmetic	*5*	Mazes	*7*		
Similarities	*6*	Geometric Design	*7*		
Comprehension	*3*	Block Design	*6*		

Developmental Test of Visual Motor Integration (Beery) AE *3 years, 10 mo.*
Wepman Test of Auditory Discrimination: Unable to follow directions to complete the test.

Testing Interpretation

Regina is a 5 year, 4 months old tiny red-haired and freckled kindergarten student. It was very difficult to test her because she was always out of her seat investigating something. She has a very short attention span for age expectations and appears to have no impulse control. The results of this testing may represent a minimal estimate of her abilities.

The overall results of the *WPPSI* indicate borderline functioning with verbal expressive skills at the lower limits of the borderline range and psychomotor skills within the borderline range. There are no significant strengths or weaknesses indicated. Relative verbal expressive strength was noted in her fund of information gleaned from school and life experiences, and in verbal concept formation. Relative weakness is noted in her ability to anticipate and judge consequences of social situations. Relative strengths in psychomotor skills at the upper limits of the borderline range include visual-motor tasks and spatial relationships.

Visual-motor integration with a written response was difficult for Regina. She tried to reproduce the geometric designs, and finally became so frustrated that she purposefully broke the pencil lead on the table. Attempts to administer the *Wepman* were unsuccessful as Regina did not understand the task required of her even after numerous examples.

In summary, Regina appears to be functioning within the borderline range of cognitive abilities in both verbal expressive and psychomotor abilities with no significant strengths or weaknesses. Relative weakness was noted in the areas of social judgment, visual-motor integration, and following directions. Short attention span and behavior interfered with performance.

School Psychologist

Developmental Evaluation

Test Administered

Carolina Developmental Profile

Testing Interpretation

Gross Motor Skills. Regina enjoyed the gross motor tasks. At first she behaved out-of-control, not following directions. She was told to return to her classroom if she did not wish to play the games. Regina was offered an M & M for each task she did correctly. This seemed to be very motivating.

Regina's overall performance was within the 5 year functioning level. She could throw a six-inch to ten-inch diameter ball at least five feet without losing balance, and throw a tennis ball using overhand throw. Regina jumped from an elevation of approximately 6 inches with both feet in the air and jumped at least two inches high from a crouched position. She walked a straight line one inch wide and ten feet long without stepping off more than three times, both forward and backward.

She walked up and down steps without support, alternating the forward foot in climbing and descending. Regina balances on one foot without support for ten seconds and balances on toes with feet together and heels off the ground for ten seconds without support. She hopped at least twice on one foot without support and jumped at least two inches high from a crouched position. Regina made a running broad jump of at least 28 inches. She experienced difficulty kicking an 8 inch ball eight feet in the air. She went too fast when trying to skip and fell down. Her overall gross motor skills appear age-appropriate.

Fine Motor Skills. Regina appears to be functioning within the five year level in fine motor skills. She can build a 3–4 block bridge and cut paper in two pieces with scissors. She can copy a circle and a square from samples; and trace a diamond pattern with a pencil. Regina can catch an 8 inch ball thrown from approximately five feet away with arms flexed. She can place 10 pennies in a box one at a time within 15 seconds. Regina can crumple a piece of paper (4½″ × 4½″) to form a ball. She experienced difficulty trying to place match sticks in a box with both hands simultaneously and could not fold a 6″ paper square to make a triangle.

Visual Perception. Regina appears to be functioning within the five year level in visual perception. She can match colors, shapes (circle, square, triangle), and animal pictures. She can name pictures of items removed from view (visual memory), and can select two identical pictures out of a set of three pictures. Regina can add parts to an incomplete man. She can put together a large 4–6 piece puzzle after demonstration. Regina could not arrange coins from largest to smallest (e.g., dime, nickel, quarter, half dollar).

Reasoning Skills. Regina appears to be functioning within the 5 year range. She discriminates big and little, long and short, bigger, slower, heavier, softly and loudly. She can count 4 blocks; state the number of wheels a bicycle has, and the number a car has. She understands first and last, but not middle. She had difficulty naming the composition of three items.

Receptive Language Skills. Regina appears to be functioning at the early 5 year level in receptive language. She can follow simple directions each containing a different preposition (e.g., under). She can select items or pictures from a small group by name, function, action, color, characteristics. Regina experienced difficulty with a 2-part direction (e.g., touch the one that is dark, but not little); and action in the future tense.

Expressive Language Skills. Regina appears to be functioning within the 4 year range in expressive language. She can name pictured objects on request and talk about the pictures. She answered comprehension questions, give purpose for having beds and TV, and give the function of eyes and ears. She can repeat a 12 or 13 syllable sentence. She has difficulty with plurals.

Social Emotional Skills. Regina is functioning within the severely deficit range in social and emotional skills. She experiences difficulty even at the 2–3 year level in social skills. She does not pay attention for 3 or 4 minutes without disturbing herself or others during a small group activity such as listening to a story. She cannot play well with other children. If she sees they have a toy that interests her she fights and takes it away. She does not play cooperatively, does not take turns, and refuses to share without becoming angry or upset. Regina does not recognize emotions in others. She does not respect others' property rights and does not participate appropriately for 10 minutes in a group activity. She seldom shows affection for other children. Regina cannot perform simple errands for teacher such as going to get paper within the classroom as she gets distracted on the way and forgets.

Summary. Regina functioned at an age-appropriate level in gross and fine motor skills, visual perception, reasoning, and receptive language in a one-to-one setting when the activities were conducted in a fast-paced game-like atmosphere with immediate rewards. In expressive language, she performed at the 4 year level. In social development, Regina's performance indicated severely delayed functioning at the 2–3 year level.

Educational Diagnostician

Pre-Academic Skills

Test Administered

Developmental Checklists for 3-, 4-, and 5-Year-Olds

Testing Interpretation

Attending. Regina experienced difficulty functioning at Level III as she cannot attend to a story 10–15 minutes or attend to an activity for 15–20 minutes. She does not have a sustained attention span for many activities.

Socializing. Regina experienced difficulty at Level IV. She does not play with peers or cooperate in classroom routines. She does not take turns and share. She does not replace materials after use and when forced to do so throws a temper tantrum screaming and kicking. Regina does not take care of her personal belongings nor respect the property of others. She is not sensitive to praise nor criticism. She does not listen and follow directions. She does not work and play cooperatively with limited supervision.

Recognizing, Discriminating, Classifying. Regina can differentiate differences in size and shape of concrete objects; classifies objects by weight (heavy, light) and by height (tall, short). She can identify eight colors. She understands same and different. She identifies and labels some spatial relationships (e.g., in/out, top/bottom). Regina can classify surfaces by texture (e.g., smooth, rough). She can name some fruits, vegetables, and meats. She appears to be functioning at the early 5 year level.

Symbolizing and Imitating. At the three year level, Regina expresses frustrations in play. She does not create imaginary playmates or engage in housekeeping as she does not hold still long enough to pretend or imitate. She does not role-play, although she is interested in the various items in the centers. She does not act out stories nor tell experiences for an experience story. She does not imitate reading behavior (e.g., turning pages front to back). This activity usually ends up with pages turned faster until torn up.

Creative Expression. Regina indicates interest in the drawing or painting center, but usually becomes angry at her inabilities and smears paint and tears up pictures. She seems interested in building with the blocks when someone else is building, but usually builds too fast so the structures fall over, then she gets angry and throws blocks. She can sing some simple songs. She functions at the 3 year level due to behavior interfering with activities.

Quantitative Concept Development. Regina appears to have mastered most of the quantitative concepts at the 3 year level. She counts by rote 1–5; understands first and last; identifies a penny, nickel, and dime; understands the concept of time (morning, night, tomorrow); recognizes basic shapes. She does not help create extended projects, form creative designs with materials or use construction materials for multiple purposes. She does not ask questions to gain information.

Social Knowledge. Regina knows her first and last names, can state her age, and follow some common directions. She does not know her parents' names, her birthday, address, or phone number.

Reading Readiness. Regina possesses only a few of the 23 skills listed in reading readiness including the following: draws circles with closed ends, connects dots with a straight line, identifies first name in print.

Summary. Regina appears to be functioning at a wide variety of levels with some significant weaknesses for age expectations. She appears to be functioning at the 3 year level in attending, socializing, symbolizing and imitating; in creative expression, quantitative concepts, and social knowledge. She appears to be functioning at the early 5 year level in recognizing, discriminating, and classifying. She possesses few reading readiness skills.

Resource Room Teacher

Classroom Observations

Regina was observed on three occasions. The first observation was early on Monday morning during "free play" at several centers. Regina could not seem to make up her mind what she wanted to do and spent 5 minutes at each of three centers. At the sand box she decided she wanted the scoop that someone else had and hit him with a toy to force him to give it to her. Teacher picked Regina up and sat her in the "naughty chair" for several minutes. She then ran to the block center and kicked over a large structure three children were cooperatively making. She ran screaming to the teacher for protection, and was placed in the "naughty chair" again.

The second observation was during recess outside. Regina did not join any of the games cooperatively. She shoved another girl out of a swing when they were all taken. She did not wait her turn on the slippery slide and rammed into another child hurting him. Much of the time she just ran wild. At the end of recess, she did not want to go back to school and threw a temper tantrum hitting, kicking, and screaming as the teacher held her by the hand pulling her toward the school. She was taken to the time-out room.

The third observation was during quiet seatwork time. The students were listening to a story and periodically they were directed to color, draw, or mark an "x" on something. Regina was unable to do this task. She marked a large X over her neighbor's paper. Regina was in constant motion even though it was a quiet-time activity. She sat on her feet, put her knees in the seat, hung over the seat, and laid on the desk. Teacher tried to ignore her.

Regina appears to be hyperactive. She is in constant motion and constantly involved in destroying peer's creations and fighting over their toys. She is tiny compared to the other kindergarten students, but easily wins any altercation because she hits, kicks, and bites with a vengeance. Her behavior is significantly interfering with her education and that of her peers. Other children try to avoid her because she is so mean.

Guidance Counselor

Evaluation Summary

Regina is a 5 year, 4 months old kindergarten student who did not attend preschool. The *WPPSI* indicates functioning within the borderline range of intelligence. Short attention span and behavior interfered with testing. Relative weakness was noted in all verbal areas especially in social judgment and following directions.

Regina appears to be motivated by primary reinforcers. She performed at the 5 year level in gross and fine motor skills, visual perception, reasoning, and receptive language. Weakness was noted in expressive language at the 4 year level. Severe deficit was noted in social behaviors at the 2–3 year level. Regina is functioning at a very immature level refusing to cooperate, take turns, or share without having a temper tantrum.

Preacademic skills testing indicates that Regina is functioning on the 3 year level in attending, socializing, symbolizing and imitating; and in creative expression, quantitative concepts, and social knowledge. She possesses few reading readiness skills. Regina appears to be functioning at the 5 year level in recognizing, discriminating, and classifying. Most developmental and preacademic skills are severe deficits for cognitive abilities.

Behaviorally, Regina is out-of-control. She does no independent school work. She lacks many of the skills important for success in kindergarten. She does not participate cooperatively, is hostile and aggressive to other children and to adults who try to control her. Her behavior is interfering with her learning and the learning of her peers.

Case Manager

DIAGNOSIS: Behavior Disordered

EVALUATION REPORT
CRAIG

Age: 7 years, 9 months
Grade: 2nd grade
Date: February , 19___

Background and Educational Concerns

Reason for Referral

Craig is a 7 year, 9 month old second grade student attending Goldberg Elementary School. His teacher has initiated this evaluation due to dramatic changes in his behavior the past four months. Craig has become quiet and withdrawn, and does not interact with other students or respond to teachers. He seems to live in a world of his own. Teacher is concerned because Craig has recently begun bringing knives to school and hides them in his desk. He may be a threat to himself and others in the classroom. This is an emergency evaluation.

Health: Immunizations are current. Physical examination indicated no specific concerns.

Vision and Hearing Screenings: Normal Range Acuities

Speech and Language Screenings

Speech screening indicates articulation, voice, and fluency are within normal limits. An informal language sample indicates that Craig speaks in grammatically correct sentences within normal limits.

Behavior History

Over the past four months, Craig has engaged in successively more deviant behaviors. He currently engages in no interpersonal relationships. When asked to join a group or play a game with a former friend, he just walks away without comment. Craig has moved his desk so that his back is to the wall and in the corner. If his desk is moved, he returns it to the wall position. Craig has gotten quite perfectionistic about his work and becomes very upset at mistakes. On some papers he erases until he makes holes in the paper. Craig has started bringing kitchen knives to school and hides them in his desk. He has never threatened anyone nor made any comments indicating that he is contemplating self-injury. However, he has marks on his arms which may be self-inflicted minor cuts.

Socio-Economic and Home Information

English is the language of the home. Craig and his 2 year old sister are the children of the owner of a small nightclub and a secretary for a finance company. They live in a settled middle class neighborhood. The children hardly ever see father, since he works at night and sleeps during the day. There appears to be no economic deprivation.

CURRENT MULTIDISCIPLINARY EVALUATIONS

This evaluation includes assessments in intelligence, perception and memory, academic achievement, social work report, and behavior evaluations.

Psychological Evaluation

Tests Administered

Wechsler Intelligence Scale for Children-Revised (WISC-R)

Verbal IQ	*107*	Performance IQ	*91*	Full Scale IQ	*99*
Information	*10*	Picture Completion	*9*		
Similarities	*10*	Picture Arrangement	*11*		
Arithmetic	*12*	Block Design	*8*		
Vocabulary	*12*	Object Assembly	*8*		
Comprehension	*8*	Coding	*8*		
Digit Span	*9*				

Testing Interpretation

Craig, a 7 year, 9 month old student, entered the testing situation somewhat anxiously. During the testing he sat rigidly, answered all questions asked, but volunteered no information.

Results of the *WISC-R* indicates overall average range cognitive functioning with average verbal expressive skills and lower limits of average psychomotor skills. There are no significant strengths or weaknesses noted. Relative strengths among verbal expressive abilities include ability to manipulate number concepts and verbal concept formation. Relative weakness, though within the average range, was noted in anticipation and judging consequences of social situations. Relative strength in psychomotor skills included the ability to recognize essential details and nonverbal judgment and planning using picture clues. Relative weakness involved the ability to learn symbols and shapes and to recreate them.

In summary, the *WISC-R* indicates that Craig's overall cognitive functioning is within the average range with average range verbal expressive and psychomotor skills. There are no significant strengths and weaknesses.

School Psychologist

Psycho-Educational Evaluation

Tests Administered

Slingerland Screening Test Form A

Far Point Copying	*Adequate*
Near Point Copying	*Adequate*
Visual Memory	*90%*
Visual Discrimination	*75%*
Visual Memory/Written Response	*85%*
Auditory Memory/Written Response	*91%*
Auditory Visual Association	*94%*

Woodcock-Johnson Psycho-Educational Battery: Tests of Cognitive Ability

Visual Perceptual Speed Cluster	GE *1.8*	AE *7-2*	%ile *26*	SS *90*
Visual Matching (92%)		Grade Range *1.5–2.0*		
Spatial Relations (94%)		Grade Range *1.5–2.0*		
Auditory Memory Cluster	GE *5.4*	AE *10-8*	%ile *89*	SS *118*
Memory for Sentences		Grade Range *3.0–6.0*		
Numbers Reversed		Grade Range *4.0–6.0*		

Woodcock-Johnson Psycho-Educational Battery: Tests of Achievement

Reading	GE *3.3*	AE *8-5*	%ile *73*	SS *109*
Word Identification		Grade Range *2.5–3.5*		
Word Attack		Grade Range *5.0–9.0*		
Passage Comprehension		Grade Range *2.5–3.5*		
Mathematics	GE *2.2*	AE *7-5*	%ile *34*	SS *94*

Calculation		Grade Range *2.0–2.5*		
Applied Problems		Grade Range *2.0–2.5*		
Written Language	GE *2.7*	AE *8-0*	%ile *63*	SS *105*
Dictation		Grade Range *2.5–3.0*		
Proofing		Grade Range *2.5–3.0*		
Punctuation and Capitalization		Grade Range *2.0–3.0*		
Spelling		Grade Range *2.0–3.0*		
Usage		Grade Range *3.0–4.0*		

Test of Written Spelling (TWS)

Grade Equivalency	*2.6*
Spelling Age	*8-0*
Spelling Quotient	*103*

Classroom Reading Inventory (Silvaroli) Listening Comprehension *5th grade*

Grade Level	*Comprehension*
3rd	*100%*
4th	*80%*
5th	*70%*

Testing Interpretation

Learning Modality. Craig's performance on the *Woodcock-Johnson* visual perceptual speed tasks indicates low-average functioning for age and cognitive expectations. On visual matching, he correctly responded to 92% of the matching numbers items, and 94% of the items attempted on the spatial relations task. His performance on auditory memory tasks indicated above average functioning for age, grade, and cognitive expectations by about three years. He correctly repeated a thirteen word sentence, and on auditory reorganization (numbers reversed), he accurately reversed a four digit number.

On the *Slingerland,* Craig's performance on near- and far-point coping indicated average range functioning for grade expectations. His far-point copying of a sentence in manuscript was neat and legible with correct punctuation and capitalization, and adequate sizing and letter formation. Improper pencil grasp appeared to interfere with smooth, flowing writing. Weakness was noted in visual discrimination due to transpositions. On the visual memory with a written response exercise, Craig demonstrated good visual memory of letter, word, and number sequences, however, he experienced difficulty in reproducing several designs reversing them. Auditory discrimination appears adequate. Craig's auditory memory with a written response revealed correctly sequenced letters, numbers and words with reversals in "d, p, 3."

Reading and Listening Comprehension. Craig's performance in reading indicated above-average functioning for age, grade, and cognitive expectations. Word identification (2.5–3.5 grade range) and passage comprehension (2.5–3.5 grade range) were within grade expectancy for age expectations. Word attack skills (5.0–9.0 grade range) were in the superior range for grade expectations. Craig's oral reading was fluent and expressive. During oral reading, he used superior phonics and structural analysis skills in decoding.

Listening comprehension (5th grade) was above-average for age, grade, and cognitive expectations. This performance indicated superior auditory memory skills. Craig's performance indicated that he experienced difficulty with inference-type questions.

Written Expression. Craig's performance on the *Woodcock-Johnson* in knowledge of written expression rules at 2.5–3.5 grade range indicates average functioning for age, grade, and cognitive expectations. Punctuation, capitalization, and spelling skills were somewhat lower at 2.0–3.0 grade range. His knowledge of verb tenses was at least one grade above expectations. Informal assessment of written composition included writing sentences. Craig wrote correctly capitalized and punctuated simple sentences. He appears to be using the written expression rules previously discussed.

Craig's performance on the *TWS* indicated average range functioning for age, grade, and cognitive expectations. He performed at the 2.6 grade level. The predictable word test is primarily phonetic and reflects Craig's superior ability in phonics skills. His performance score was somewhat depressed by letter reversals.

Mathematics. Craig's performance in mathematics indicates functioning in the average range for age, grade, and cognitive expectations. On the calculation subtest, he correctly computed a double digit subtraction problem without regrouping. He does not appear to know the algorithms of subtractions with regrouping, multiplication, or division. The applied problems test performance revealed good reasoning skills. Craig understands the concepts of addition and subtraction. He correctly calculated a multiplication problem by reasoning and computing on his fingers. Though Craig utilizes visual clues, he appears to compute abstractly.

Summary. Craig does not appear to have any processing deficits severely impacting on his academic functioning. The auditory channel appears to be the strongest mode for learning (above-average), while the visual mode appears average. He occasionally reverses and transposes letters and numbers.

Academically, Craig's skills all appear to be in the average range for age, grade, and cognitive expectations. Of concern, however, is Craig's awkward left-handed pencil grasp and the limitations it appears to put on his writing performance in terms of volume and neatness. This is not a severe problem now, but a concern with potential to be a severe problem soon.

Educational Diagnostician

Social Worker Report

Mother and grandmother were consulted regarding Craig's behavior changes at school within the past several months and the teacher's concerns. Mother reported that over the past year quarrels between Craig's father and her about his coming home from the bar drunk have become more and more violent. Just prior to the Court Injunction and Legal Separation, Craig saw his father beat and severely injure his mother. Neighbors called the police. Mother was taken in the ambulance to the hospital and father was handcuffed and taken to jail in the police car. The neighbor stayed with the children until the grandparents arrived the next day and took them to the grandparents' home. After mother was released from the hospital, Craig and his sister returned home with her.

Father has threatened to kidnap the children if mother divorces him. Mother feels that was "the alcohol talking." Father has entered a drug/alcohol treatment program which will soon begin family counseling.

Mother indicated that Craig was traumatized by the situation. Little sister was asleep during the "event" so does not seem to be having adjustment problems. Craig is afraid of father and if mother mentions his name, Craig begins to sob and beg "no." Mother has found kitchen knives hidden under Craig's pillow and when she questioned him about it he responded that they were "for protection." Mother was not aware that he had taken knives to school. Mother began to cry softly and asked, "What should we do?"

The following recommendations were made to mother:

(1) Consult family physician for physical examination and consultation.
(2) Consult family counselor at the drug program.
(3) School guidance counselor will begin crisis intervention.

School Social Worker

Behavior Evaluation

Test Administered

Behavior Evaluation Scale

Subscales	*Standard Scores*	*Quotients*
1. Learning Problems	9	95
2. Interpersonal Difficulties	4	70
3. Inappropriate Behavior	5	75
4. Unhappiness/Depression	4	70
5. Physical Symptoms/Fears	3	65

Testing Interpretation

Results of the *Behavior Evaluation Scale* indicate that Craig is currently functioning significantly different from his average peers in Interpersonal Difficulties, Inappropriate Behavior, Unhappiness/Depression, and Physical Symptoms/Fears. Currently, Craig appears to have an inability to maintain the previously satisfactory interpersonal relationships with peers and teachers. He has become very withdrawn and does not interact with peers at recess or in the classroom. He is not usually rude, he just does not seem to notice that anyone is trying to interact with him.

Craig engages in inappropriate types of behaviors or feelings under normal circumstances. He has physically and emotionally withdrawn from others in the classroom. He has moved his desk away from others with his back to the wall with full view of all who come into the classroom or who walk by it. He has kitchen knives hidden in his desk.

Craig has a general pervasive mood of unhappiness or depression. Previously, he exhibited a quick wit and saw humor in many situations. He has excellent verbal skills and contributed frequently in class. Currently, he never smiles and seems to have "built an invisible box around his emotions." His eyes no longer sparkle with mischief. Craig appears to have developed fears regarding personal problems. This is accentuated by placing himself and his desk in a watchful, defensive position and bringing weapons to school. He does not appear to be afraid of anyone currently at school.

Teacher writes page numbers of assignments on the board and Craig attempts to complete these assignments, but does not interact with the teacher or peers. No one seems to exist.

Guidance Counselor

Evaluation Summary

Craig is a 7 year, 9 months old second grade student who was referred due to significant behavior changes. His overall intellectual functioning appears to be within the average range with average range verbal expressive and psychomotor abilities. No true strengths or weaknesses were noted. The auditory channel appears to be the strongest for learning with above average skills, however, visual processing skills appear to be within the average range. Craig still reverses and transposes some letters and numerals.

Academically, all skills appear to be within the average range for age, grade, and cognitive expectations. The major academic concern is his awkward left-handed pencil grasp and the limitations it puts on his writing performance in terms of completing long written assignments.

The social worker indicates that the family has been in a state of crisis. Father currently is receiving alcohol abuse rehabilitation and the family will soon begin family counseling as part of that process. Craig has been traumatized and is so fearful of father that he hides knives under his pillow and brings them to school. Behaviorally, Craig is currently functioning significantly differently from his average peers in interpersonal relationships, inappropriate behavior, unhappiness and depression, and fears. He has become very withdrawn and unhappy. He has postured his desk in a defensive position and brought knives to school "for protection" from father. Currently, he does not seem to be a danger to other students as he seems unaware of their existence.

Case Manager

DIAGNOSIS: Behavior Disordered

RE-EVALUATION REPORT
GARY

Age: 12 years, 8 months
Grade: Ungraded Middle School
Date: May , 19___

Background and Educational Concerns

Reason for Referral

Gary, a 12 year, 8 months old student labeled behavior disordered, attends an ungraded alternative middle school for severely behavior disordered students. His classroom teacher has requested a special re-evaluation to consider mainstreaming Gary into a regular Junior High School based on his age/grade appropriate academic skills. He has been in special classrooms for behavior disordered students for the past five years and teacher thinks returning to a "normal" school would serve as incentive to control his behavior.

Health

School health records indicate that immunizations are current. Recent physical examination indicated no concerns.

Vision and Hearing Screenings

Screenings indicated normal range visual and auditory acuities.

Speech and Language Screenings

Speech and language appear to be within normal limits.

Behavioral History

Gary was originally diagnosed behavior disordered in the second grade. Although he displayed no academic problems (as indicated by individual testing), his behavior was out-of-control. Gary exhibited 0% task focus, short attention span, very distractible, and constantly on-the-move. He was violent and aggressive toward peers and teacher: hitting, biting, scratching, kicking, cursing. He refused to stay in his seat, and would leave the classroom without permission wandering about the halls or outdoors to the playground. He set a fire in the boys bathroom wastebasket on two occasions. On one occasion he smeared the walls in the bathroom and himself with his own feces.

After diagnosis, Gary was placed in a self-contained classroom with seven other behavior disordered boys. Gary was prescribed ritalin by the family physician and his behavior improved, somewhat. He responded well to immediate reinforcement behavior management. Gary was programmed individually in academics and moved at his own pace. Over the next four years, each time efforts were made to mainstream Gary into a regular classroom situation he behaved aggressively to students and teachers. During attempts to mainstream Gary into the music class he tore up the teacher's music, banged uncontrollably on the piano, and broke several rhythm band instruments. On an attempt to mainstream him into math class he broke the rulers to be used in the measurement assignment, hit other students, and tore up several math books.

Currently, Gary attends an ungraded alternative middle school. Academically, he has performed well there on individualized programming. At the beginning of each week, he and the teacher decide how much work should be accomplished in each academic area each day and write a contract. Gary then schedules his own day including academics and rewards (e.g., Atari, computer games, etc.). In order to watch the Friday afternoon movie, however, Gary must have completed his contract. Gary works well under this system with "Nobody telling me what to do."

Socio-Economic and Home Information

Gary is the youngest of three sons of a "biker." The family lives on the edge of town in a small poorly tended house. Father and two older sons, all high school dropouts, operate a motorcycle repair shop out of the garage. The yard and shop are full of motorcycles. Each family member owns his own bike. Their neighborhood and the "hangouts" the family attends are involved with this alternative life style. They, also, dress the role. Periodically, Gary comes to school "beaten up" from "getting mouthy with my old man." School authorities seldom contact the parents due to their aggressiveness and threats toward school officials.

CURRENT MULTIDISCIPLINARY EVALUATION

This evaluation includes the following assessments: intelligence, perception and memory, academic achievement, behavior, and social skills.

Psychological Evaluation

Test Administered

Wechsler Intelligence Scale for Children-Revised (WISC–R)

Verbal IQ	*97*	Performance IQ	*115*	Full Scale IQ	*105*
Information	*7*	Picture Completion	*10*		
Similarities	*10*	Picture Arrangement	*13*		
Arithmetic	*10*	Block Design	*13*		
Vocabulary	*10*	Object Assembly	*15*		
Comprehension	*11*	Coding	*10*		
Digit Span	*9*				

Testing Interpretation

Gary, a 12 year, 8 months old student at the alternative middle school, arrived at the testing center accompanied by his teacher who indicated that he would receive "special rewards" for appropriate behavior. When his teacher left he said, "I've done this before, so I may get bored and need a break. I'll let you know. Let's get this show on the road." Gary completed the testing, sitting backwards straddling the chair, but without any behaviorial difficulties.

Results of the *WISC–R* indicate overall cognitive functioning within the average range with average range verbal expressive skills and psychomotor skills at the upper limits of the high average range. Little variability was noted among the verbal expressive scores. Gary's weakest performance, lower limits of low average range, was in information gained from experience and education. He demonstrated average range abilities in practical knowledge and social judgment, ability to manipulate number concepts, ability to see relationships between facts and ideas, and auditory sequencing.

Gary demonstrated average to superior range psychomotor skills. His performance revealed average range ability in recognizing essential details and in speed of visual-motor reaction and association of symbols. He evidenced high average to superior abilities in nonverbal judgment and visual-motor perception and coordination. Gary performed within the superior range in visual-motor coordination and assembly tasks.

In summary, Gary's intellectual functioning appears to be within the average range with average range verbal skills and high average to superior psychomotor skills. His behavior was appropriate with promised "rewards" by the teacher. As he completed each task, he went quickly to the next task without unnecessary conversation. At the end of the testing, he swung his leg over the chair to stand up, gave a half-salute, and left.

School Psychologist

Psycho-Educational Evaluation

Tests Administered

Malcomesius Screening Test

Far Point Copying	*100%*
Near Point Copying	*100%*
Visual Memory	*94%*
Visual Discrimination	*100%*
Visual Memory/Written Response	*92% items/83% sequencing*
Auditory Memory/Written Response	*82% items/100% sequencing*
Auditory Discrimination	*100%*

Woodcock-Johnson Psycho-Educational Battery: Tests of Cognitive Ability

Visual Perceptual Speed	GE *7.4*	AE *12-6*	%ile *47*	SS *99*
Visual Matching (95%)		Grade Range *6.0–8.0*		
Spatial Relations (96% items, 91% puzzles)		Grade Range *8.0–12.9*		
Auditory Memory	GE *12.9*	AE *29*	%ile *92*	SS *121*
Memory for Sentences		Grade Range *3.0–7.0*		
Numbers Reversed		Grade Range *12.9*		

Woodcock-Johnson Psycho-Educational Battery: Tests of Achievement

Reading		GE *8.5*	AE *13-8*	%ile *57*	SS *103*
	Subtests	*Grade Ranges*			
	Word Identification	*7.0–9.0*			
	Word Attack	*7.0–12.9*			
	Antonyms-Synonyms	*6.0–9.0*			
	Analogies	*9.0–12.9*			
	Passage Comprehension	*7.0–11.0*			
Mathematics		GE *7.6*	AE *12-11*	%ile *55*	SS *102*
	Subtests	*Grade Ranges*			
	Quantitative Concepts	*7.0–11.0*			
	Calculation	*7.0–9.0*			
	Applied Problems	*7.0–9.0*			

Illinois State Dept. of Education Secondary Informal Reading Inventory

Listening Comprehension	9th grade	*80%*
	10th grade	*75%*
	11th grade	*60%*

Test of Written Language (TOWL): Written Language Quotient *85*

Vocabulary	%ile *2*	SS *69*
Thematic Maturity	%ile *25*	SS *90*
Spelling	%ile *37*	SS *95*
Word Usage	%ile *50*	SS *100*
Style	%ile *37*	SS *95*

Testing Interpretation

Learning Modality. On the *Malcomesius,* Gary's performance was age and grade appropriate. He experienced no significant difficulties in auditory or visual processing tasks with or without a written response. Gary performed within or above age and grade expectations on the *Woodcock-Johnson* visual perceptual tasks. He correctly answered 95% of the visual matching of numbers items, and 91% of the spatial relations puzzles performing significantly above grade expectations. On the auditory memory tasks, Gary performed within the superior range, however, there was a significant difference between subtests with memory for sentences at the 3.0–7.0 grade range, while numbers reversed was at the 12.9 grade range. All primary learning modalities appear to be strong with no significant weakness.

Reading and Listening Comprehension. Gary's overall performance in reading indicated average range functioning for age, grade, and cognitive expectations. Basic reading skills of word identification, word attack, synonyms and antonyms, and analogies; and passage comprehension appear equally well developed with no significant weaknesses. Gary's oral reading was fluent. He utilized his knowledge of phonics and syllabication skills in decoding unfamiliar words. He utilized context clues effectively in decoding unfamiliar words and in deriving meaning. No areas of deficiency were revealed by the testing.

Gary's performance indicates above-average listening comprehension for age, grade, and cognitive expectations. At the 9th grade level, he experienced difficulty with vocabulary definition. At the 11th grade level, he experienced difficulty with vocabulary definition and inference questions.

Written Expression. Gary's performance in written language indicated below-average functioning for age, grade, and cognitive expectations. His performance in spelling indicated average functioning for age, grade, and cognitive expectations. At the higher levels he experienced short-vowel substitution errors. Performance on the Word Usage subtest indicates average functioning. His primary area of difficulty was verb tenses. He appears to understand plurals, comparatives, and pronoun antecedents. Gary's performance on the Style subtest (capitalization and punctuation) revealed average functioning. Major areas of deficit included inconsistency in performance, use of apostrophes, use of commas and quotation marks.

Gary's use of higher level vocabulary words in his expressive writing sample was in the severely deficit range for cognitive expectations. He utilized only one higher level vocabulary word. His performance on the Thematic Maturity subtest (story content and structure) was in the low average range for cognitive expectations. Though, he attempted to write an integrated story using the stimulus pictures, the events in the story appear unrelated. Informal assessment of the written language sample indicated that he utilized his knowledge of capitalization and punctuation, wrote in complete sentences, but did not write an integrated story.

Mathematics. Gary's overall performance in mathematics at the 7.6 GE indicates functioning in the average range for age, grade, and cognitive expectations. No primary areas of deficit were evident. He understood quantitative concepts, calculation, and applied problems. He appears to understand the algorithms of addition, subtraction, multiplication, and division. He appears to know basic mathematics facts of addition, subtraction, multiplication, and division. Gary did, however, experience difficulty calculating fractions.

On the applied problems subtest his performance revealed good abstract mental calculation skills and good abstract reasoning ability. He revealed understanding of computation of two-step problems and demonstrated good ability to calculate problems dealing with money, time, and measurement. Gary revealed the ability to sort through extraneous information to isolate basic information required to solve problems and revealed understanding of relationship concepts that indicate which mathematical process is required in problem-solving. Gary experienced difficulty calculating applied problems dealing with fractions.

Summary. Gary does not appear to be experiencing processing deficits. Both auditory and visual channels in isolation and integrated with a written response appear to be good methods of learning. Auditory sequencing (e.g., reorganization of numbers) is an excellent skill area.

Academically, Gary appears to be functioning commensurate with cognitive expectations in reading, math, spelling, and mechanics areas of written language. Utilization of higher level vocabulary and content of story writing appear to be weaknesses.

Educational Diagnostician

Behavior Evaluation

Test Administered

Behavior Evaluation Scale

Subtests	*Standard Scores*
1. Learning Problems	*70*
2. Interpersonal Difficulties	*65*
3. Inappropriate Behavior	*65*
4. Unhappiness/Depression	*95*
5. Physical Symptoms/Fear	*100*
Behavior Quotient	*71*

Testing Interpretation

The *Behavior Evaluation Scale* was completed by Gary's teachers at the Alternative Middle School. Currently, Gary is on a behavior management plan that allows him to control scheduling his academic work periods and give input in determining the amount of work he will complete on contract. This type of arrangement is possible in this alternative school environment. The *BES* was completed based on Gary's usual behavior not on the program.

Gary's overall behavior appears significantly different from peers in the areas of learning problems, interpersonal difficulties, and inappropriate behavior. His learning problems are directly related to interfering behavior. His current academic progress appears appropriate for cognitive expectations. However, when not allowed to manage his own academic program he continuously refuses to begin tasks, refuses to complete class assignments or homework, and does not follow directions (oral or written).

In the area of Interpersonal Difficulties, Gary appears to be severely disordered. He does not interact appropriately with any peers or faculty. Generally, he is verbally and physically abusive to peers. He makes derogatory comments, curses continually, verbally threatens peers and teachers. He always seems very angry and very immature in that he always wants his own way. Gary does not appear to have any friends at school. Most students provide him a large amount of personal space.

Gary appears severely behavior disordered in the area of inappropriate behavior. Continuously throughout the day, he uses obscene or profane language typical to the "biker" group. Daily at various times he exhibits the following behaviors: (1) off-task behaviors, (2) fails to participate verbally or physically in group situations, (3) demonstrates sudden or dramatic mood changes, (4) acts impulsively without apparent self-control. He continuously fails to consider the consequences of his behavior refusing to obey teachers' directives or classroom rules, and talks at inappropriate times.

Gary does not appear to be unhappy or depressed. He appears to gain satisfaction from intimidating and bullying until he gets his own way. His family prescribes to a "counter culture" in which force and aggression are rewarded behaviors. He periodically throws temper tantrums, but these appear designed to stimulate fear in peers and teachers and force compliance with his preferences. Gary does not exhibit a tendency to develop physical symptoms or fears associated with personal or school problems.

Comment. The change in Gary's behavior when allowed to contract his academic work and self-schedule as compared to his behavior in traditional small groups is so dramatic as to speculate that much of his deviant behavior is purposeful and self-controllable. He has sabotaged mainstreaming efforts and appears to prefer the alternative school situation. This is understandable as his family lives an alternative life style. It is my opinion that Gary will continue to thwart efforts to mainstream him into a rigid academic setting.

School Counselor

Social and Emotional Development (Informal Assessment)

Using informal assessment and observation, Gary appears severely deficit in social and emotional development compared to same-aged peers.

Social Perspective-Taking. Social perspective-taking is an area of severe deficit for Gary. He does not show concern about how others feel or express concern for others at school. He does not appear to be developing insight into the reciprocal nature of social interactions. He does not appear to engage in social communication and use the information to modify his behavior in various settings.

Social Regulation and Moral Development. Gary experiences severe deficits in the area of social regulation and moral development. He does not conform to several sets of rules regarding moral codes and behaviors. He has learned one set of rules and behaviors and uses those regardless of how inappropriate in all situations. He does not change his behavior based on the social responses of others. Gary has not learned through indirect socialization techniques and has not increased his ability to get along with people. He does not regulate his own behavior according to social rules. He does not understand that appropriate behavior differs in various social settings.

Social Problem-Solving. Social problem-solving is an area of significant deficit. Gary is not sensitive to social problems and social consequences. He uses verbal and physical intimidation to solve any problems he experiences.

Interactions with Peers. Gary does not interact appropriately with peers in supervised or unsupervised school activities. He wears his "biker" attire in all situations. Friendship does not appear very important to him. He does have several followers who fear him yet admire his toughness. Gary is not learning self-control in staying out of trouble. He does not negotiate or apologize unless he receives immediate reinforcement or personal benefit. His social and emotional behavior appears tied to his "biker" image.

In summary, Gary appears severely deficit in social perspective-taking, social regulation and moral development, social problem-solving, and peer social relationships.

School Social Worker

Evaluation Summary

Gary is a 12 year, 8 month old student who was originally diagnosed behavior disordered in the 2nd grade. Current cognitive functioning appears to be within the average range with average range verbal expressive skills and high average to superior psychomotor skills. He has excellent visual-motor skills. Both the auditory and visual channels with oral or written response are good channels for learning.

Academically, Gary is performing within cognitive expectations or higher in reading (basic skills and comprehension at 8.5 GE), mathematics (calculation, and reasoning at 7.6 GE), and the written expression mechanics of spelling, word usage, capitalization and punctuation. Listening comprehension is an area of significant strength at the 10th grade level. Gary experienced difficulty in the expressive writing sample in using higher level vocabulary and with story content and structure.

Gary's behavior evaluation indicates severely discrepant behavior in the learning situation, interpersonal problems, and inappropriate behavior. He is primarily concerned with using verbal and physical force and intimidation to do things "his way." As long as he controls the situation, he remains calm. He has sabotaged every attempt to mainstream back into regular school classes and appears to prefer the alternative school situation. The social development evaluation indicated that Gary is severely deficit in social perspective-taking, social regulation and moral development, social problem-solving, and peer social relationships.

Case Manager

DIAGNOSIS: Behavior Disordered

EVALUATION REPORT
DANIEL

Age: 15 years, 5 months
Grade: Ungraded Alternative High School
Date: July , 19___

Background and Educational Concerns

Reason for Referral

Daniel is a 15 year, 5 months old student attending the ungraded high school at a Boys Residential Center where he currently lives due to Juvenile Court placement. This special referral was requested by his teachers due to his superior academic functioning, and to consider mainstreaming him to the local high school for classes.

Health

School health records indicate immunizations are current. Recent physical examination indicated no medical concerns.

Vision and Hearing Screenings: Normal Range Acuities

Speech and Language Screenings: Within Normal Limits

Behavioral History

Daniel was removed from his home and placed in the Boys Residential Center by the Juvenile Court for extreme rebellion, disobedience, delinquency, and truancy. He quit attending school, refused to obey his parents, and began running with a gang. The first time he was arrested for slashing tires and breaking store windows, he was given one year probation because his role in the activity was not clear. Daniel's older brother appears to be a leader in the gang. Daniel broke probation by not attending school, and was arrested when he took a car and went "joy riding."

Before dropping out of school, Daniel had never been a discipline problem. He was somewhat shy. He had always made good grades, completed his work and homework, and was obedient to teachers.

Socio-Economic and Home Information

Daniel's step-father is an American aircraft engineer. His mother is Vietnamese, and works in an oriental restaurant. His parents were married when he was three years old. He has no information about his American father who abandoned them when living near an Army Post. The family lives in a middle class neighborhood. Though mother speaks English with an accent, Daniel does not. Daniel's older brother has "been a problem" since elementary school days. The parents feel that Daniel's recent rebellion is due to influences of his older brother. There is no economic deprivation.

CURRENT MULTIDISCIPLINARY EVALUATION

This evaluation includes assessments in intelligence, perception and memory, academic achievement, behavior evaluation, and classroom demands.

Psychological Evaluation

Test Administered

Wechsler Intelligence Scale for Children-Revised (WISC-R)

Verbal IQ	*115*	Performance IQ	*130*	Full Scale IQ	*123*
Information	*13*	Picture Completion	*16*		
Similarities	*12*	Picture Arrangement	*14*		
Arithmetic	*14*	Block Design	*16*		
Vocabulary	*12*	Object Assembly	*15*		
Comprehension	*13*	Coding	*15*		

Testing Interpretation

Daniel is a 15 year, 5 months old ungraded high school student attending classes at the Residential Center school. He entered the testing situation somewhat shyly, but was socially appropriate and indicated that he was ready for the testing.

Results of the *WISC-R* revealed a nonsignificant discrepancy between superior range verbal expressive skills and gifted range psychomotor skills. The Full Scale IQ is in the superior range. Daniel's overall potential is assumed to be within the gifted range. His performance revealed high average skills in relaying information from education, in using practical knowledge and social judgment, in verbal concept formation, and in the quality of language used. He performed within the superior range in concentration and arithmetic reasoning, and the ability to manipulate number concepts.

Psychomotor skills are an area of significant strength with scores within the gifted range. Superior skills were demonstrated in ability to recognize essential details and visual-motor coordination in assembly tasks. Daniel performed in the gifted range in visual-motor perception and coordination involving analysis and reproduction of abstract designs. Superior range performance was noted in nonverbal judgment using picture cues, and speed of visual-motor reaction and association of symbols.

In summary, Daniel's potential appears to be within the gifted range with superior range verbal expressive skills and gifted range psychomotor skills. Visual-motor integration is an area of superior ability.

School Psychologist

Psycho-Educational Evaluation

Tests Administered

Woodcock-Johnson Psycho-Educational Battery: Tests of Cognitive Ability

Verbal Perceptual Speed	GE *12.9*	AE *25*	%ile *76*	SS *111*
Visual Matching (100%)		Grade Range *12.9*		
Spatial Relations (92% items, 87% puzzles)		Grade Range *8.0–12.9*		
Auditory Memory	GE *12.9*	AE *36*	%ile *90*	SS *119*
Memory for Sentences		Grade Range *10.0–12.9*		
Numbers Reversed		Grade Range *12.9*		

Illinois State Dept. of Education Secondary Informal Reading Inventory

Listening Comprehension	10th grade	*100%*
	11th grade	*95%*
	12th grade	*90%*

Woodcock-Johnson Psycho-Educational Battery: Tests of Achievement

Reading	GE *12.9*	AE *23*	%ile *80*	SS *113*

Word Identification	Grade Range *10.0–12.9*			
Word Attack	Grade Range *12.9+*			
Passage Comprehension	Grade Range *11.0–12.9*			
Synonyms and Antonyms	Grade Range *11.0–12.9*			
Analogies	Grade Range *12.0+*			
Mathematics GE *12.9*	AE *32*	%ile *92*	SS *121*	
Quantitative Concepts	Grade Range *12.9+*			
Calculation	Grade Range *12.9+*			
Applied Problems	Grade Range *12.9+*			

Wide Range Achievement Test-Revised (Spelling) GE *9.3* %ile *70* SS *108*

Test of Written Language: Written Language Quotient *110*

Vocabulary	%ile *75*	SS *110*
Thematic Maturity	%ile *75*	SS *110*
Word Usage	%ile *90*	SS *120*
Style	%ile *25*	SS *90*

Testing Interpretation

Testing Behavioral Observations. Rapport was readily established. Daniel conscientiously attempted the tasks presented and worked diligently throughout the testing period. He was polite and socially appropriate. He was not verbally spontaneous, but he politely responded to all questions asked and all social comments made in getting acquainted. Daniel seemed rather quiet and shy by nature and did not make much eye contact. He appeared to enjoy the challenge of the testing. The results of the testing appear to be valid assessments of Daniel's current functioning level.

Learning Modality. Daniel's performance indicates excellent visual learning modality skills. Visual perceptual speed skills involving number discrimination and spatial relationships were significant strengths. His performance reveals superior auditory learning modality skills. Short-term auditory memory for sentences is an area of strength. Daniel showed superior ability in the area of auditory reorganization and sequencing of numbers.

Reading and Listening Comprehension. Daniel's performance in reading indicates above-average functioning for age expectations. He appears to have no weaknesses in the area of reading. Word attack skills and analogies are areas of strength. Daniel's oral reading was fluent and he utilized his knowledge of phonics, syllabication, and context clues in decoding unfamiliar words and in deriving meaning. On more difficult passages, Daniel indicated a preference for oral reading as an aid to comprehension.

Listening comprehension at the 12th grade level and above is an area of strength for age and grade expectations. At the 12th grade level, he experienced difficulty with the vocabulary definition questions.

Written Expression. Daniel's performance in written language indicated above-average functioning for age expectations. Performance on the Word Usage subtest indicates superior functioning in verb tenses, comparatives, and irregularly formed plurals. His performance on the Style subtest (capitalization and punctuation) revealed low average functioning. There were no major areas of deficit. His performance reflected minor errors (e.g., forgetting to capitalize the first letter of a quotation). He possesses good capitalization and punctuation skills.

Daniel's performance in spelling indicated above-average functioning for age expectations. He utilizes his good visual memory and phonics skills. On more difficult words he committed substitutions and omissions of similar sounding vowels and consonants.

Daniel's use of high level vocabulary words in his expressive writing sample was in the above-average range. He utilized 28 higher level vocabulary words including "prospered, incredibly, acquaintances." His performance on the Thematic Maturity subtest (story content and structure) was in the above-average range. Daniel's creative story reflects the ability to integrate historical events with fantasy to create a story of the future. Informal assessment of the written language sample indicated that he wrote in complete sentences. He wrote an integrated story utilizing his knowledge of capitalization and punctuation. He did not, however, write in paragraphs. He experienced some difficulties with verb tenses and word endings.

Mathematics. Daniel's overall performance in mathematics indicates functioning in the superior range for age expectations. He appears to experience no significant difficulties in mathematics. He understands the algorithms of addition, subtraction, multiplication, and division. He correctly computed problems dealing with decimals, fractions, and algebraic equations.

On the applied problems subtest his performance revealed good abstract calculation skills. He demonstrated strengths in abstract reasoning ability. He revealed understanding of relationship concepts that indicate which mathematical process is required in problem-solving. His performance revealed understanding of computation of two-step problems; calculation of money, time, and measurement. Daniel's performance revealed the ability to sort through extraneous information to isolate basic information required to solve problems. He experienced difficulty with problems dealing with probability and statistics.

Summary. Daniel does not appear to be experiencing any learning deficits. Auditory and visual learning skills appear to be in the superior range. Academically, his performance indicates above-average to superior range functioning for age expectations. He appears to be functioning in the above-average range in reading, spelling, and written language; and in the superior range in mathematics.

Educational Diagnostician

Behavior Evaluation

Test Administered

Behavior Evaluation Scale

Category Subtests	*Standard Scores*
1. Learning Problems	*115*
2. Interpersonal Difficulties	*95*
3. Inappropriate Behavior	*100*
4. Unhappiness/Depression	*100*
5. Physical Symptoms/Fear	*100*
Behavior Quotient	*103*

Testing Interpretation

The *Behavior Evaluation Scale* was completed by Daniel's teacher at the Boys Residential Center School. Daniel's overall behavior rating is within the average range as are the scores for each individual subtest. The evaluation indicates that he does not have specific behavior problems interfering with his learning. Daniel does not display interpersonal difficulties or inappropriate behaviors in the classroom. He is respectful of peers and adults. Though he does not talk a lot he is not afraid to voice his opinion. Daniel is respected by his classmates and he is often selected to help solve problems. He does not demonstrate unhappiness or depression nor indicate physical symptoms and irrational fears.

In summary, Daniel's classroom behavior falls within the average range with no specific concerns indicated.

School Counselor

Classroom Demands Assessments

Informal Tests Administered

Classroom Demands Interview	*Excellent*
Interview on Essay Project/Report Writing	*Excellent*
Checklist for Assessing Student's Examinations	*Excellent*
Checklist for Assessing Student's Notebook	*Excellent*
Gaining Information from Tests (Interview)	*Excellent*

Testing Interpretation

Due to mainstreaming considerations involved with Daniel's evaluation, a number of informal assessments were administered to get a better idea of his chances for success in the public high school. His overall abilities as a student appear to be excellent.

Daniel was given the *Classroom Demands Interview Record Form* on which he had to complete two columns for each of his classes: Classroom Demands and Evaluation Procedures. He was directed to write down the classroom demands or learning activities that he had to do in each specific teacher's classroom in order to be successful (e.g., take lecture notes, write lab report, read text). In the second column he was directed to write down the procedures each teacher would use in evaluating his success and giving a grade (e.g., essay tests, multiple choice tests, notebook, term paper). Daniel appeared to have a very good grasp of what he needed to do to be successful in each class and exactly what the teacher expected.

One of his recent papers was selected for evaluation using the *Interview Questions on Essay Project/Report Writing.* Daniel had a very good grasp of the assignment. He indicated his planning and research strategies, his writing techniques (e.g., outline, rough drafts, preparation of final copy), and self-evaluation (e.g., grade he felt he deserved on the paper). Daniel is quite well organized and has a specific system for writing reports and essays.

Daniel completed the *Checklist for Assessing Student's Examinations.* He indicated his specific strategy for studying for a test, and specific test taking behavior. A recent test was secured from one of his teachers and evaluated for the quality of product submitted (e.g., handwriting, written composition mechanics, relevance of answers). Daniel was able to do the task very well, indicating a well planned strategy for test taking.

A *Checklist for Assessing Student's Notebook* was used to evaluate Daniel's Literature Journal. He evaluated it for overall organization, handwriting, and content. Since the Journal is an ongoing "free thought" exercise there was not a specific organization required. He was asked what he thought his teacher expected and how the notebook would be graded. Daniel appeared to have a good understanding of the demands of this task, although in his present situation he is not often asked to prepare a notebook.

Daniel completed the *Gaining Information from Text* form. From analyzing his responses he appears to have good study strategies: refers to figures and illustrations, reads the headings, and underlines or takes notes on specific items that he wants to remember specifically. Daniel appears to have excellent study skills and a good concept of himself as an active learner.

Resource Room Teacher

Evaluation Summary

Daniel is a 15 year 5 months old bilingual Vietnamese-American student attending an alternative high school at a Boys' Residential Center. Current psychological evaluation indicates that Daniel's potential is in the gifted range (psychomotor skills) with superior range verbal expressive skills. He appears to have superior range visual and auditory processing skills with an oral or written response.

Academically, Daniel is performing within the above-average to superior range in all academic areas functioning at least at the 12th grade level. Mathematics is an area of superior ability. According to the informal classroom demands assessments, Daniel understands what he must do to be successful in the classroom. He knows what is expected by teachers when assigning an essay, report, or notebook. He understands how to efficiently gain information from a text and to prepare for a test. Daniel understands his role as a student.

Within the classroom, Daniel demonstrates appropriate student behaviors. He does not appear to have interpersonal difficulties or learning problems. Daniel does not exhibit extreme unhappiness, fear, depression, or physical symptoms. Within the classroom, his behavior is appropriate.

Daniel's inappropriate behaviors within the community and truancy which resulted in adjudication as a delinquent adolescent are not problems in the Residential Center. His inappropriate behaviors were not transferred to the classroom at the Residential Center.

Case Manager

DIAGNOSIS: Gifted

Chapter Six

CASES OF LEARNING DISABLED STUDENTS

A student is considered to have a specific learning disability if s/he does not achieve at the proper age and ability levels when provided appropriate learning experiences, and demonstrates a severe discrepancy between intellectual ability and achievement in one or more of the following areas: oral expression, listening comprehension, written expression, basic reading skills, reading comprehension, mathematics calculation, mathematics reasoning and/or preacademic skills (Federal Register, Dec. 29, 1977). The IQ range of learning disabled students may vary from functioning just above the mental retardation cut off (IQs 70–75) through gifted ranges.

Preschool Age/Grade: Diana
Primary Age/Grade: Drew
Intermediate Age/Grade: Erica
Secondary Age/Grade: Michelle

EVALUATION REPORT
DIANA

Age: 5 years, 9 months
Grade: Kindergarten
Date: October , 19___

Background and Educational Concerns

Reason for Referral

Diana is a 5 year, 9 month old kindergarten student at Adams Street Elementary School. She was referred for evaluation by her kindergarten teacher because of academic failure. She is unable to work independently, and has a very short attention span.

Diana has numerous academic deficits. She does not know her alphabet or recognize letters, does not recognize numerals, cannot listen and comprehend, cannot follow directions, cannot do any of the pre-academic work of her classmates. Diana is easily distracted and attempts to interact with peers while they are working independently or in a group situation. The teacher aide has been assigned to work almost exclusively with Diana in a one-to-one situation to prevent classroom disruptions.

Health

No medical history or immunization data is available. Diana's mother has 30 days to show proof of immunizations according to state law or Diana will be terminated from school. The school social worker has been contacted.

Vision and Hearing Screenings: Normal Range Acuities

Speech and Language Screenings

Diana exhibited maturational articulation deficits. Her performance indicated deficits in language development areas including names for concepts and associative responses. A language evaluation is recommended.

Behavior History

Diana's behavior problems appear to be a result of immaturity and short attention span rather than rebellion and intent to challenge authority figures. She talks or sings almost continuously, and remains in her seat for only minutes at a time. Diana cannot work independently on any school work.

Socio-Economic and Home Information

English is the language of the home. Diana, her mother, and two younger sisters live in a small three bedroom house with her aunt (mother's sister) and 3 cousins. All six children range in age from 2–7 years old. Diana indicated that the children fight a lot and must be sent to their rooms. She indicated that they sleep in sleeping ("fleeping") bags on the beds.

Diana misses quite a bit of school, by her report, she must stay home and take care of her younger sisters. She frequently comes to school wearing urine-smelling clothing, apparently Diana and her sisters sleep together and the youngest one wets the bed. Diana often comes to school hungry.

There is no telephone and mother does not respond to notes sent home. The school security officer was sent to the home to deliver a letter regarding the referral for special education testing. Mother indicated an interest, but did not understand the problem. Social services was contacted.

CURRENT MULTIDISCIPLINARY EVALUATION

This evaluation includes assessments in intelligence, perception and memory, academic achievement, communication, and social development.

Psychological Evaluation

Tests Administered

Peabody Picture Vocabulary Test-Revised (PPVT-R) IQ 81
Stanford-Binet Intelligence Scale (Form L–M) IQ 86
Boehm Test of Basic Concepts 55 %ile using Low SES Norms
Human Figure Drawing Low Average to Average Range
Test of Visual-Motor Integration 5 years, 7 mo./44th %ile

Testing Interpretation

On the *Stanford-Binet,* Diana's overall performance fell within the low average range of intelligence. All items were passed (basal) at Level V, partial success was achieved at Level VI, and all items were failed (ceiling) at Level VII. Diana's performance on the *PPVT-R* indicated low average language and cognitive functioning.

Diana successfully completed several visual-motor tasks including completing a partial drawing, and copying a simple geometric figure. She was unable to successfully complete several mazes. Perceptual-motor assessment indicated average development for age expectations in terms of ability to perceive and reproduce geometric designs.

Diana's *Human Figure Drawing* was examined according to the Koppitz criteria. Her drawing consisted of a head, eyes, nose, mouth, ears, hair, arms, and legs. One expected item, a trunk, was not included. This performance suggested intellectual functioning within the low average to average range, and, as such, is commensurate with obtained measured intellectual data.

Diana correctly identified 29 of 55 concepts presented on the *Boehm.* This performance placed her at the 55th %ile (using low socio-economic norms). She correctly identified "top," "second"; but could not identify such concepts as "next to," "almost," "least."

In summary, Diana is a 5 year, 9 months old kindergarten student functioning within the low average range of intelligence.

School Psychologist

Communication Evaluation (Informal Assessment)

Receptively, Diana appears to be functioning at the 3 to 3½ year developmental level. She points to pictures of some common objects when they are named and can identify some objects when told their use. She experiences difficulty answering the "wh-questions" because she wants to tell a story or relate any associative information that comes to mind. She understands negatives "no, not, can't, don't." Due to short attention span, she does not listen to usual children's stories read aloud. She cannot carry out a series of 2–4 related directions. She needs directions specified one direction at a time. Diana has some understanding of comparatives.

Expressively, Diana is functioning on the 3–4 year developmental level. Her expressive language is significantly affected by her deprived environment, lack of basic concepts, and lack of labels for concepts. She uses sentences of three or more words and talks about past experiences. At school she has learned some nursery rhymes and to sing abc's from watching Sesame Street. Her speech is understandable to strangers, though she makes some maturational misarticulations such as "fl" for "sl" (e.g., fleeping for sleeping).

In summary, Diana appears to be functioning receptively and expressively at the 3–4 year developmental level in language.

Speech/Language Pathologist

Psycho-Educational Evaluation

Tests Administered

Woodcock-Johnson Psycho-Educational Battery: Tests of Achievement

PreSchool Cluster	GE *1.0*[1]	AE *4-0*	%ile *3*	SS *70*
Knowledge	GE *1.0*[2]	AE *3-6*	%ile *2*	SS *69*

Slingerland Screening Test: PreReading, Revised

Far Point Copying	*88%*
Visual Discrimination	*38%*
Visual Memory to Written (symbols)	*70%*
Auditory Visual Association-Pictured Object	*75%*
Letter Knowledge and Sound Symbol	*0%*

Developmental Tasks for Kindergarten Readiness (DTKR)

Subtests	*Norm Rating*	*Percent Accuracy*
Social Interaction	*D*	*70*
Name Printing		*80 (Dana)*
Body Concepts: Awareness	*C*	*63*
Body Concepts: Use	*D*	*20*
Auditory Sequencing	*A*	*83*
Auditory Association	*D*	*38*
Visual Association	*D*	*0*
Visual Motor	*B*	*81*
Visual Memory	*C*	*14*
Color Naming	*A*	*100*
Relational Concepts	*C*	*60*
Number Knowledge: Counting	*A*	*100*
Number Knowledge: Use	*B*	*75*
Number Knowledge: Naming	*D*	*10*
Alphabet Knowledge	*D*	*4*

Test of Early Reading (TERA)

Total Raw Score	*6*
Reading Quotient	*73*
Percentile	*3*
Reading Age	*3-7*

Testing Interpretation

Testing Behaviors. Diana is a very verbal five year, nine month old kindergarten student. Her continuous talking appeared to interfere with her concentration and task performance. Her attention span appears to be only a few minutes at most even in a one-to-one structured setting. She was very pleasant and eager to make friends with the examiner.

Diana's thinking was very associative. Any stimulus item would remind her of something that she just had to talk about or a song to sing. It was difficult to refocus her attention on task, to stop the singing, or to cease the story before she was finished. She did not remain in her seat longer than a few minutes at a time. She could be encouraged to do a task by offering a Mickey Mouse pencil for proper behavior. She demonstrated no independent work skills.

Learning Modality. Several subtests of the *Slingerland* were administered to assess auditory and visual processing. Diana wrote some letters of her first name (DANA). Her performance on the far-point copying test was adequate, however, she required much reinforcement and redirection to complete the task. She experienced significant difficulties on the visual discrimination of letters task making two transpositions of letters, two inversions, and four letter reversals. Visual discrimination appears to be an area of significant weakness. On the visual memory with written response subtest, Diana performed in the below average range. On two items she forgot one detail each, she indicated to the examiner that she remembered something but could not remember where to put it. Diana's performance on the auditory-visual association task indicated low average functioning. Her attention had to be continually redirected to the task.

Several subtests of the *DTKR* concerned learning modality processing. No clear learning modality preference emerged. Diana's performance in visual motor skills indicated functioning in the average range for age expectations. Auditory sequencing was an area of strength. Areas of severe deficit included visual discrimination, visual memory, and auditory association. On the visual discrimination subtest, Diana missed all items by reversing, inverting, or substituting letters. On the visual memory subtest, she accurately answered only one item, committing reversals and transpositions. Diana's performance on the auditory association subtest indicated that she talked associatively about the stimulus, but seldom answered the question asked.

Kindergarten Readiness Skills. Diana demonstrated strengths in color naming and rote counting skills. Her performance in number use indicated functioning in the average range for age expectations. However, Diana's performance indicated deficits in body awareness and relational concepts; and severe deficits in knowledge of body use, social interactions, number naming, and alphabet knowledge. Diana appears to have no number-symbol association knowledge. She only recognizes two alphabet letters and has not yet acquired letter-symbol association.

On the Preschool Cluster of the *Woodcock-Johnson,* Diana's performance indicated that knowledge of preschool skills is an area of severe deficiency for age expectations. She performed approximately two years below expectancy. Diana could identify no letters, answered three applied problems (picture clues), and wrote the letter "O." On the Knowledge Cluster, her performance indicated functioning 2½ years below age expectations. Diana could not identify animals or the sounds associated with them, tell why she went to school ("to be quiet"), or relate nursery rhymes.

On the *TERA,* Diana's performance indicated functioning approximately 2½ years deficit for age expectancy. She recognized the McDonald's symbol and that of the 7 Eleven Store. She could point to the top and bottom of a page. She answered a question correctly after being read a short story, and sang her alphabet. She identified no letters or words correctly.

Summary. Diana appears to be severely deficit in the visual memory and visual discrimination processing areas. She, also, experiences difficulties with auditory association. Areas of adequate performance include the following: far-point copying, visual memory to written (symbols), auditory visual association (pictured object), auditory sequencing, and visual motor tasks.

Academically, Diana's performance indicates functioning in the severe deficit range for age expectations in all areas. She recognizes no numbers or letters, though she can count by rote and recite her alphabet. She appears deficit by 2½ years in general knowledge information. She knows her colors and understands one-to-one correspondence to seven.

Educational Diagnostician

Social Development (Informal Assessment)

Diana is socially immature. She has little idea of the purpose of school. She talks continuously, eager to make friends. She shows affection for her younger siblings and is expected to care for them when mother is gone. She does not appear to be able to interpret adults' emotions from facial expressions and intonation. She is eager to please but because of her short attention span and lack of knowledge of the purpose of school her behaviors are inconsistent.

Diana is unable to play simple table games because she does not possess many of the readiness skills used in the games—colors, numbers, alphabet letters, relational concepts. She does not understand games with rules. Socially, Diana is functioning at approximately the 3 to 3½ year level.

Resource Room Teacher

Evaluation Summary

Diana is a 5 year, 9 months old kindergarten student. Her overall cognitive ability falls within the low-average range of intelligence (IQ 86). She lacks understanding of many of the basic cognitive concepts required to perform mathematics tasks (e.g., least, almost). Psychomotor skills of perceiving and reproducing geometric designs are within average expectations, as is auditory sequencing. Diana experienced significant difficulties with visual discrimination, visual memory, and auditory association. Thus, no clear learning modality preference emerges as she experiences problems with both visual and auditory processing skills.

Academically, Diana has not mastered preschool skills. While she can rote count, she has no understanding of one-to-one correspondence above seven and no number-symbol association knowledge. Diana is functioning 2½ years deficit in general preschool knowledge and in reading readiness skills. She possesses no sound-symbol letter knowledge.

Behaviorally, while not severely behavior disordered, her short attention span and continuous talking significantly interfere with acquisition of basic skills. Her inability to monitor her own behavior and to change it to be more appropriate in the school setting causes her to experience difficulty with the teacher. She is frequently punished for misbehavior and has no concept of what she did incorrectly or why the teacher is mean to her. Socially, Diana is functioning at the 3 to 3½ years developmental level.

Diana appears to live in an environmentally deprived home and has not been exposed to relational concepts and language expected for her age. She appears to lack an understanding of the purpose of school and her role as a student. While a child of Diana's measured ability level would be expected to function approximately a year below her chronological age expectations, after nearly one year of kindergarten Diana appears to be functioning 2½ to 3½ years below expected developmental levels.

Case Manager

DIAGNOSIS: Learning Disabled (Preacademic Skills, Oral Language)

EVALUATION REPORT
DREW

Age: 7 years, 9 months
Grade: 2nd grade
Date: December , 19____

Background and Educational Concerns

Reason for Referral

Drew is a 7 year, 9 months old second grade student attending Washington Elementary School. The primary reasons for the school's request to have Drew evaluated include short attention span, significant problems with any writing task (e.g., copying work from the board and/or textbook), and problems with mathematics. Teachers indicate that he seems bright.

Drew is functioning in the lower third of his class in all academic areas. He received failing grades in mathematics, spelling, and language the second grading period. Behaviorally, Drew gets along well with peers and adults. He appears rather shy, but has a good sense of humor.

Health

Drew's immunizations are current. An intramural physical examination indicated no medical concerns. He has a history of ear infections and seasonal allergy problems for which he takes dimetapp or sudafed.

Speech and Language Screenings: Within Normal Limits

Vision and Hearing Screenings

School screenings indicate adequate visual (with glasses) and auditory acuities.

Behavior History

In the classroom Drew is somewhat shy. His attention span is short and he seems tired after concentrating for a brief period. He has several "buddies" with whom he has been friends since preschool days, and who appreciate his subtle humor. He works well in a small group, particularly with his "buddies".

Socio-Economic and Home Information

English is the language of the home. Drew is the only child of professional parents, an accountant and a broker. The family lives in a new upper-middle class suburban housing area, just down the block from Drew's "buddies." There are no obvious social or economic environmental concerns.

Drew's parents keep him busy in intramural sports, Boy Scouts, and summer league activities. They enjoy Sunday afternoon "family activities." Drew has an entertainment center in his interconnecting playroom and bedroom, and unlimited toys and games which he enjoys playing with his friends. Drew does have several regular chores—emptying the waste baskets into appropriate recycling bins in the garage, making his bed, picking up his toys before he goes to bed, and keeping his room tidy. He is supervised by the housekeeper until his parents get home from work.

CURRENT MULTIDISCIPLINARY EVALUATION

This evaluation includes assessments in the areas of intelligence, perception and memory, academic achievement, and social development.

Psychological Evaluation

Tests Administered

Wechsler Intelligence Scale for Children-Revised (WISC–R)

Verbal IQ	*101*	Performance IQ	*91*	Full Scale IQ	*97*
Information	*10*	Picture Completion	*10*		
Similarities	*13*	Picture Arrangement	*11*		
Arithmetic	*10*	Block Design	*7*		
Vocabulary	*11*	Object Assembly	*8*		
Comprehension	*12*	Coding	*7*		
Digit Span	*6*	Mazes	*7*		

Peabody Picture Vocabulary Test-Revised (PPVT–R) AE *8-3* SS *111*
Test of Visual Motor Integration (Beery) AE *6-0*

Testing Interpretation

Drew is a delightful seven year, nine months old second grade student. He is rather shy, but rapport was easily established. Drew conscientiously attempted every task presented, however, he tired easily during the performance subtests. He indicated that his glasses were new and he was not used to them as yet.

Results of the *WISC–R* indicate Drew's overall cognitive functioning is within the average range. Verbal expressive skills were within the average range, while psychomotor skills were within the lower limits of the average range. Relative strengths in verbal expressive skills were noted in verbal concept formation, practical knowledge and social judgment. A significant weakness was noted in auditory sequencing of numbers. Psychomotor skills involving visual-motor perception and coordination of space relationships and symbols, and the ability to learn symbols and recreate them were difficult for Drew. He also experienced difficulty with tasks requiring visual planning and following a visual pattern.

The results of the *PPVT–R* indicated that Drew functioned above age expectations in receptive language. On the *Beery,* Drew experienced significant difficulties functioning 1½ years deficit for age expectations in observing and reproducing shapes. Difficulties were consistent with his functioning on the psychomotor skills of the *WISC–R.*

In summary, Drew's overall cognitive functioning is within the average range with weaknesses in visual-motor skills and spatial relationships. Receptive language appears to be an area of strength.

School Psychologist

Psycho-Educational Evaluation

Tests Administered

Woodcock-Johnson Psycho-Educational Battery: Tests of Achievement

Reading Cluster	GE *2.5*	AE *7-8*	%ile *46*	SS *98*
Mathematics	GE *2.0*	AE *7-2*	%ile *22*	SS *88*
Written Expression	GE *2.2*	AE *7-8*	%ile *43*	SS *97*

Slingerland Screening Test Form B

Far Point Copying	*poor*
Near Point Copying	*poor*
Visual Memory	*92%*
Visual Discrimination	*75%*
Visual Memory to Written	*33%*

Auditory Memory to Written	*poor*
Auditory Discrimination	*94%*
Auditory Visual Association	*72%*

Woodcock-Johnson Psycho-Educational Battery: Tests of Cognitive Ability

Visual Perceptual Speed Cluster	CA *7-9*	AE *6-10*	GE *1.6*	%ile *17*	SS *86*
Visual Matching	Grade Range *1.0–1.5*				
Spatial Relationships	Grade Range *1.5–2.0*				
Auditory Memory Cluster	CA *7-9*	AE *9-0*	GE *4.0*	%ile *89*	SS *118*
Memory for Sentences	Grade Range *12.9*				
Numbers Reversed	Grade Range *1.0–2.0*				

Test of Written Spelling (TWS): GE *1.3* SA *6-7* SQ *84*

Test of Written Language (TOWL): Written Language Quotient *90*

Vocabulary	%ile *5*	SS *75*
Thematic Maturity	%ile *25*	SS *90*
Word Usage	%ile *25*	SS *90*
Style	%ile *63*	SS *105*

Durrell Analysis of Reading Difficulties Listening Comprehension *5th grade*

Informal Reading Inventory (Silvaroli) Form D

Oral Reading	Word Recognition	Comprehension
1st grade	Independent	*80%*
2nd grade	Frustration	*80%*
3rd grade	Frustration	*20%*

Testing Interpretation

Learning Modality. Several instruments were administered to assess Drew's auditory and visual processing skills. On the *Woodcock-Johnson,* his performance on visual speed tasks indicated functioning in the below average range for age expectations. Both visual matching of numbers and spatial relationships were difficult for him.

Drew's performance on auditory memory tasks indicated above average functioning for age expectations. Auditory memory subtest scores, however, reveal a significant discrepancy among skills. On the memory for sentences task, Drew scored at the 12.9 grade range, while on the numbers reversed task he scored at the 1.0–2.0 grade range. Drew's performance indicates excellent immediate auditory recall for words, but poor auditory reorganization skills especially with numbers.

On the *Slingerland,* Drew experienced considerable difficulties with both near-point and far-point copying. Drew's performance on the visual memory test was very good, but he drew lines to assist in visual tracking which seemed to be very difficult. Though visual discrimination performance was adequate, he experienced three letter transpositions (self-corrected one). Drew experienced significant disabilities on the visual memory to written task including following the directions, spatial organization, letter and number reversals, substitutions, omissions, transpositions, additions, and inversions.

Though Drew's auditory discrimination skills are good, he experienced difficulty in organizing his page (following directions), transposing numbers, and reversing letters. Auditory memory to written tasks presented significant difficulties for Drew including all of the previously mentioned problems associated with a written task. Auditory visual association is nearly adequate, however, responses indicate that he is drawing lines to assist with visual tracking and experiences many letter transpositions.

Reading and Listening Comprehension. Drew's overall performance in reading indicated average range functioning for age, grade, and cognitive expectations. On the *Silvaroli,* Drew's performance indicated oral reading word recognition instructional level at the 1st grade level. At the 2nd grade level he mispronounced two words and omitted eight words, and at the 3rd grade level he mispronounced 3 words and omitted 23 of the 105 words in the passage. He read quickly and omitted the words without a pause in reading. Word recognition appears to be an area of significant weakness. Comprehension is an area of relative strength. Despite orally reading at frustration level at the 2nd grade level, his comprehension was well within instructional level.

Listening performance on the *Durrell* indicated instructional level at the 5th grade level. On the comprehension check he scored 80% indicating excellent listening skills especially on areas of interest to him.

Written Expression. Deficiency areas in manuscript writing indicated on the *Slingerland* included sizing, spatial organization, spacing, and letter formation. In writing words he committed the following errors: letter additions, transpositions, substitutions, and letter omissions. The *TWS* performance indicates functioning in the below-average range for age and grade expectations in spelling. Drew's score was depressed due to reversals. He performed one year below age and grade expectations on the predictable (phonetic) words and could spell none of the unpredictable (nonphonetic) words. Spelling appears to be an area of significant weakness.

Drew's performance in written language (knowledge of rules) on the *Woodcock-Johnson* indicated average range functioning for age and grade expectations, however, a significant discrepancy exists among the subscores. On punctuation, capitalization, and word usage, Drew scored in the 3rd grade range, while in spelling his scores were at the 1.5 grade level.

On the *TOWL,* Drew's overall performance indicates average range functioning for age expectations, though significant discrepancies exist among the subtests. Drew demonstrated above average knowledge of punctuation and capitalization rules, but he did not utilize those rules in his expressive writing sample. On word usage, Drew performed above-average in verb tenses, plurals, and comparatives. On the expressive writing sample, Drew's performance was in the low average range in thematic maturity and significantly below average range in use of higher level vocabulary. Informal evaluation reveals that Drew did not write an integrated story, but rather, described the pictures. He did not write in complete sentences, nor utilize proper punctuation and capitalization. Drew's thoughts were connected by the use of conjunctions.

Mathematics. Drew's performance in mathematics indicated below average functioning for age and grade expectations. Calculation scores were at the 1.5–2.0 grade range, while applied problems was at the 2.5 grade range. He experienced significant difficulty with calculation in addition and subtraction. He has not mastered the basic math facts, experienced difficulty with alignment of numbers, and experienced difficulty with the algorithms. He cannot regroup in addition or subtraction, and experienced difficulty with money, time, and fractions. Applied problems were a relative strength for Drew in areas of numerical reasoning, mental calculation, and word problems.

Summary. Drew experienced strengths and significant disabilities in both the auditory and the visual learning modes. Auditory and visual memory in isolation were areas of strength, but became significant weaknesses when paired with a written response. Visual discrimination deficits among letters and numbers are significantly impacting his academic functioning. He experiences difficulty with following directions, spatial organization, visual tracking, and very simple visual-motor tasks. Drew is experiencing extreme perceptual integration deficits.

Academically, Drew's perceptual integration deficits seem to be negatively impacting his skill acquisition in reading word recognition, mathematics calculation, and all expressive writing tasks. Academics that depend on reasoning such as reading and listening comprehension, and mathematics reasoning reveal above grade level functioning.

Educational Diagnostician

Social Development (Behavioral Observation)

An informal social development assessment indicated that Drew was functioning at the 8 year old developmental level. He is friendly, selective in his choice of friends, and has several "best buddies." He likes organized games in small groups, but also enjoys team sports. Drew uses language as his medium of interaction. He understands the peer group norms of his social strata. He has a good sense of humor.

Emotionally, Drew is sensitive to the feelings of others especially his buddies. He is sensitive to criticism and ridicule, and is quite concerned about his academic failure. He is happy much of the time and secure in many areas. Drew is, however, beginning to feel insecure about school now that written expression takes precedence over oral language.

Resource Room Teacher

Evaluation Summary

Drew is a 7 year, 9 months old second grade student. Current psychological evaluation indicates average range cognitive functioning with average verbal skills and low average psychomotor skills. Drew experienced significant difficulty on visual-motor and visual discrimination skills, and spatial relationships. Auditory memory tasks with a written response also presented significant difficulties.

Academic assessment in reading indicates significant weakness in word recognition (1st grade level) and strength in reading comprehension (2nd grade level). Listening comprehension is an area of significant strength (5th grade level). On written composition skills of knowledge of capitalization, punctuation, and word usage in isolation, Drew functioned within the average range. On the written expression creative writing sample, Drew did not use these composition skills accurately. He experienced significant difficulty with handwriting and in story construction. Spelling is an area of significant weakness. Drew's math performance appears to be an area of weakness with a significant difference between his abilities in calculation and applied problems. Drew's perceptual motor problems especially visual processing problems significantly interfered with his academic functioning in areas that require visual discrimination, visual memory, and visual memory with a written response.

Social development and behavior appear to be areas of strength. Language skills in social communication and humor are areas of strength. Drew is feeling some concerns regarding his academic failure.

Case Manager

DIAGNOSIS: Learning Disabled (basic reading skills, math calculation, and written expression)

EVALUATION REPORT
ERICA

Age: 12 years, 5 months
Grade: 6th Grade
Date: April , 19___

Background and Educational Concerns

Reason for Referral

Erica is a 12 year, 5 months old 6th grade student at Eisenhower Elementary School. Teachers indicate that Erica seems to be intelligent, yet she experiences significant difficulties in reading and written expression. Her grades in mathematics are excellent, but she often makes minimum passing grades in content area subjects requiring a lot of reading and written papers.

This evaluation was initiated by Erica's parents due to her medical diagnosis of Tourette syndrome and the increased symptoms exhibited this school year. Parents want the teachers at the Junior High School to be prepared for Erica's handicapping condition to facilitate her acceptance there.

Health

School records indicate that Erica's immunizations are current. A school sports physical last August indicated no specific concerns.

Medical records indicate a diagnosis of Tourette syndrome. Erica takes haldol to help control the TS symptoms but she experiences fatigue and problems with concentration as side effects. Facial tics (e.g., eye blink, nose twitch, grimaces) began last school year. The symptoms have increased and this school year she has experienced involuntary head jerks, tongue thrusts, foot stomping, and verbal ticks of grunting and barking. Erica is quite bewildered and embarrassed by this situation and is receiving counseling.

Vision and Hearing Screenings: Adequate visual and auditory acuities.

Speech and Language Screenings

School screenings indicate that speech and language skills are within age expectations. Erica is verbally spontaneous, has a superior vocabulary, and speaks in grammatically correct sentences.

Behavior History

Teachers report that Erica's behavior has been appropriate for age expectations, however, there appears to be a direct relationship between increased TS symptoms and withdrawal. She continues to show respect for peers and authority figures. When others tease or laugh about the TS symptoms she is exhibiting, she cries. At present her controllable behavioral responses are not severe enough to be considered behavior disordered.

Socio-Economic and Home Information

English is the language of the home. Erica is the only child of theatrical parents who own and operate a prosperous dinner theatre. Parents frequently appear in the plays performed at the theatre. In the past Erica has also taken part in these theatrical productions. She has taken tap and ballet lessons for six years and plays a flute in the elementary school band. The family lives in a renovated Victorian house in the older section of town where mostly older couples live. There appears to be no economic deprivation.

MULTIDISCIPLINARY EVALUATION

This evaluation includes assessments in intelligence, perception and memory, academic achievement, and social/behavioral development.

Psychological Evaluation

Test Administered

Wechsler Intelligence Scale for Children-Revised (WISC–R)

Verbal IQ	*120*	Performance IQ	*130*	Full Scale IQ	*128*
Information	*14*	Picture Completion	*14*		
Similarities	*14*	Picture Arrangement	*13*		
Arithmetic	*13*	Block Design	*15*		
Vocabulary	*12*	Object Assembly	*17*		
Comprehension	*14*	Coding	*12*		
Digit Span	*13*				

Testing Interpretation

Erica is a 12 year, 5 months old 6th grade student, who entered the testing situation shyly but politely. She was friendly and well-mannered. Rapport was readily established and she worked diligently throughout the testing. She discussed the problems associated with Tourette syndrome.

Results of the *WISC-R* indicate that overall cognitive abilities fall within the upper limits of the superior range with superior range verbal expressive skills and psychomotor skills within the gifted range. Erica's performance indicates an excellent command of the English language both receptively and expressively. She demonstrates superior verbal concept formation and higher-level thinking skills in social problem-solving.

There are no true weaknesses among the psychomotor skills which range from high average to gifted. Spatial relationships are a definite strength. A significant strength is Erica's ability to see the relationship of parts to wholes, and logical insight into space relationships. Relative weakness is noted in the ability to learn symbols and shapes and to recreate them.

In summary, Erica's performance on the *WISC-R* indicates intellectual functioning within the upper limits of the superior range with superior range verbal skills and gifted range psychomotor skills.

School Psychologist

Psycho-Educational Evaluation

Tests Administered

Malcomesius Screening Test

Far Point Copying	*Good*
Near Point Copying	*Good*
Visual Memory	*88%*
Visual Discrimination	*100%*
Visual Memory/Written Response	*90% Sequencing/80% Items*
Auditory Memory/Written Response	*100% Sequencing/82% Items*

Woodcock-Johnson Psycho-Educational Battery: Tests of Cognitive Ability

Visual Perceptual Speed Cluster	GE *9.0*	%ile *70*	SS *108*

Visual Matching		Grade Range *7.0–8.0*		
Spatial Relations		Grade Range *11.9–12.9*		
Auditory Memory Cluster		GE *11.9*	%ile *99*	SS *135*
Memory for Sentences		Grade Range *11.9*		
Numbers Reversed		Grade Range *11.9*		

Woodcock-Johnson Psycho-Educational Battery: Tests of Achievement

Reading	GE *4.4*	AE *9-7*	%ile *21*	SS *88*
Word Identification		Grade Range *5.0–6.0*		
Word Attack		Grade Range *3.5–5.0*		
Passage Comprehension		Grade Range *3.5–5.0*		
Mathematics	GE *8.0*	AE *13-5*	%ile *71*	SS *108*
Calculation		Grade Range *9.0–11.9*		
Applied Problems		Grade Range *7.0–9.0*		
Written Language	GE *11.9*	AE *18-10*	%ile *91*	SS *120*
Dictation		Grade Range *3.5–5.0*		
Proofing		Grade Range *7.0–11.0*		
Punctuation and Capitalization		Grade Range *10.0–11.9*		
Spelling		Grade Range *3.5–4.5*		
Usage		Grade Range *8.0–11.0*		

Test of Written Language Written Language Quotient *90*

Vocabulary	%ile *5*	SS *75*
Thematic Maturity	%ile *75*	SS *110*
Word Usage	%ile *16*	SS *85*
Style	%ile *50*	SS *100*

Classroom Reading Inventory (Silvaroli): Listening Comprehension

Levels	Listening Comprehension
8	*100%*
9	*90%*
10	*80%*

Illinois State Depart. of Education Secondary Informal Reading Inventory

Levels	Listening Comprehension
11	*80%*

Testing Interpretation

Learning Modality. Erica's performance on the *Woodcock-Johnson* visual perceptual speed tasks indicate above-average functioning for age and grade expectations, but significantly below cognitive expectations. On the visual number matching task, she accurately responded to every item attempted, correctly discriminating four digit numbers, and functioning at the 7.0–9.0 grade range. On the spatial relations subtest, Erica performed at the 11.9 grade range, accurately responding to 91% of the items attempted and 90% of the puzzles.

Erica's performance on auditory memory tasks at the 11.9 grade range indicates superior range functioning for age, grade, and cognitive expectations. Her excellent memory for sentences (11.9 grade range) indicates remembering up to 15 word sentences. Her performance on the auditory reorganization task (numbers reversed) indicates accurately reversing 7 digits and functioning at the 11.9 grade range.

Subtests of the *Malcomesius* were administered to assess processing on classroom-like tasks in 6th, 7th, and 8th grades. The results of visual and auditory tasks indicated excellent information processing skills with verbal oral or written responses. All number and letter sequences were accurate, although there were some spelling errors.

Reading and Listening Comprehension. Erica's performance on the *Woodcock-Johnson* reading test indicated significantly deficit functioning for age, grade, and cognitive functioning. Her overall reading performance at the 4.4 GE indicates a 2 year deficit for age and grade expectations. Her performance on the word attack subtest (3.5–5.0 grade range) indicates gaps in knowledge. She tends to substitute short vowel sounds; experienced difficulties with double vowels, sounds of "y," and silent letters. Erica appears to understand basic syllabication rules. She read fluently through the 3rd grade level basal. At higher levels her performance indicated that she did not use phonics or syllabication as major decoding strategies, but appeared to rely on word configuration and context clues. Passage comprehension (3.5–5.0 grade range) appears to be a significant deficit also.

Listening comprehension at the 11th grade level appears to be an area of significant strength commensurate with cognitive expectations. On the *Silvaroli,* Erica answered 100% of the questions correctly at the 8th grade level, 90% at the 9th grade level, and 80% at the 10th grade level. On the *Illinois,* she answered 80% of the questions at the 11th grade level, experiencing difficulty with questions requiring sequencing of events and vocabulary definitions. A significant difference exists among superior listening comprehension skills (11th grade) and significantly deficit reading functioning (GE 4.4).

Mathematics. Erica's overall performance in mathematics (GE 8.0) on the *Woodcock-Johnson* indicates above-average functioning for age and grade expectations, but below cognitive expectations. On the calculation subtest (9.0–11.9 grade range), Erica performed at least three years above grade level expectations. She understands the basic mathematical algorithms including fractions; and the basic facts and utilizes them in computation.

On the applied problems subtest (7.0–9.0 grade range), she performed 1–3 years above grade level expectations. Erica appears to have a good understanding of the computation of two-step problems. She experienced difficulty with problems involving time, percentages, and fractions. Erica has a very good reasoning ability and very good skills in abstract calculation.

Written Expression. On the *Woodcock-Johnson,* Erica's overall performance was significantly above age and grade expectations but commensurate with cognitive expectations. However, there is a wide performance range among subskills. Spelling (3.5–5.0 grade range) appears to be an area of significant weakness, and clearly affected by her weak word attack skills (3.5–5.0 grade range). Dictation was significantly weak as well due to the spelling requirement. The writing mechanics skills of proofing, punctuation and capitalization, and word usage in isolation appear to be significantly above grade level expectations.

Erica was administered the *TOWL* to assess application of knowledge of written language rules. Her overall performance indicated low-average functioning for age and grade expectations, but severely deficit for cognitive expectations. Her performance indicated age-appropriate ability to capitalize and punctuate practice sentences and paragraphs. However, comparison with the results of the *Woodcock-Johnson* indicates a greater ability to proof sentences for incorrect capitalization and punctuation errors than to utilize this skill during composition.

On the *TOWL* word usage subtest, Erica's performance indicates an area of severe deficit functioning for age, grade, and cognitive expectations. She experienced difficulty utilizing correct verb tenses, irregularly formed plurals, and pronoun antecedents. This represents a significant discrepancy when compared to performance on the *Woodcock-Johnson* indicating that Erica appears to have a much better ability to recognize a word usage error than to apply correct word usage skills during composition.

The vocabulary and thematic maturity subtest scores on the *TOWL* were determined by analyzing her creative writing sample. Erica performed in the severe deficit range for age, grade, and cognitive expectations in usage of higher level vocabulary in her creative writing sample. Her performance on thematic maturity was commensurate with her verbal cognitive expectations. Informal analysis revealed that Erica wrote an integrated story utilizing the three stimulus pictures. She wrote in paragraphs using correctly capitalized and punctuated sentences, but incorrect verb tenses and spelling errors. Her story incorporated pictorial relationships, reasons for environmental hostility, original names for spacelings, and the role of the spacelings.

Summary. Erica does not appear to have a significant processing deficit at this time. Auditory memory skills appear superior even for cognitive expectations. Visual memory skills are average for age and grade expectations. She experienced some difficulty in the area of visual discrimination, however, performance was age-appropriate.

Academically, Erica experiences significant intraindividual differences with scores ranging from superior to severely deficit for cognitive expectations. Areas of strength include listening comprehension, mathematics, and mechanics of written expression. Areas of significant weakness include reading, basic skills and comprehension; spelling; and written composition (word usage and usage of higher level vocabulary).

Educational Diagnostician

Classroom Observation

Test Administered

Informal Behavioral Observation

Testing Interpretation

Erica was observed informally on three separate occasions over a one week period. She was observed during reading group in the morning, at noon recess, and during an afternoon study period. During these observations her behavior socially and as a student were appropriate. In the classroom she was on-task and actively involved with completing her assigned tasks. She worked diligently until the tasks were completed during group teacher-directed activities and independently. At the noon recess period, she sat with a small group of girls socially talking. Her behavior seemed appropriate.

Although during these observation periods, Erica did not exhibit any Tourette syndrome symptoms, this teacher has observed the TS symptoms on other occasions. During these occasions, Erica became quite upset, began crying, and had to be taken to the school nurse's office.

Resource Room Teacher

Evaluation Summary

Erica is a 12 year, 5 month old 6th grade student who was diagnosed last summer by her physician as having Tourette syndrome. Cognitively, Erica is functioning within the upper limits of the superior range (FSIQ 128) with superior verbal skills (VIQ 120) and gifted range psychomotor skills (PIQ 130). She does not appear to be experiencing any information processing deficits. Both auditory and visual channels are good for learning with an oral or a written response. Auditory skills are significant strengths.

Academically, Erica shows wide intraindividual differences from significantly deficit to superior for cognitive expectations. Listening comprehension (11th grade) is a significant strength, while reading comprehension (3.5–5.0 grade range) and reading skills (3.5–5.0 grade range) are significant weaknesses. Math calculation (9.0–11.9 grade range) and reasoning (7.0–9.0 grade range) are strengths for age and grade expectations. Spelling is an area of significant weakness. Ability to proofread and discover written mechanics errors is significantly better than the ability to use those skills in a written composition. Word usage and the use of higher level vocabulary words in written expression are significant weaknesses, while thematic maturity is a strength. Informal analysis of written composition indicated good basic structure (e.g., sentences and paragraphs), and correct use of capitalization and punctuation.

Behavior observations indicate appropriate social and student behaviors, unless experiencing TS symptoms, at which time she becomes frightened and embarrassed and cries.

Case Manager

DIAGNOSIS: Gifted/Learning Disabled (Reading basic skills, reading comprehension, and written expression) and Other Health Impaired (Tourette syndrome)

RE-EVALUATION REPORT
MICHELLE

Age: 14 years, 0 months
Grade: 8th
Date: May , 19___

Background and Educational Concerns

Reason for Referral

Michelle is a 14 year, 0 months old student just completing the 8th grade. She was diagnosed learning disabled in reading and written expression at the end of 5th grade. She is enrolled in regular classes and receives daily Resource Room assistance at the Junior High School. Currently, Michelle is failing English, science, social studies, and is receiving a C− in mathematics. This is a routine re-evaluation to determine appropriate programming at the High School.

Health

Immunizations are current. Michelle's last physical examination before school started indicated no specific concerns. She periodically misses school due to severe sinus headaches and takes prescribed medication as needed.

Vision and Hearing Screenings

School vision and hearing screenings indicate normal functioning.

Speech and Language Screenings

Speech and language screenings indicate normal functioning.

Behavior History

Michelle's classroom behavior is generally appropriate. During lectures she experiences great frustration and questions neighbors about the notes they are taking or tries to copy their notes, thus, missing more of the lecture. Teachers feel that she does not pay attention in class.

Socio-Economic and Home Information

English is the language of the home. Michelle is the youngest of three daughters of a barber (father) and a real estate agent (mother). The parents just bought a new home in a new middle class subdivision. Michelle's sisters are in high school and do not experience difficulties in school. Michelle has always had trouble in school. She has an after school babysitting job for two primary grade children until their parents get home from work. Michelle regularly attends several organizations and her church youth group. There appears to be no economic deprivation.

CURRENT MULTIDISCIPLINARY EVALUATION

This evaluation includes the following assessments: intelligence, perception and memory, academic achievement, social development, and vocational assessment.

Psychological Evaluation

Tests Administered

Wechsler Intelligence Scale for Children-Revised (WISC-R)

Verbal IQ	*94*	Performance IQ	*109*	Full Scale IQ	*101*
Information	*10*	Picture Completion	*12*		
Similarities	*9*	Picture Arrangement	*11*		
Arithmetic	*9*	Block Design	*12*		
Vocabulary	*10*	Object Assembly	*12*		
Comprehension	*9*	Coding	*9*		
Digit Span	*7*				

Testing Interpretation

Michelle is an attractive 14 year, 0 month old eighth grade student who came to the testing somewhat reluctantly. Rapport was established readily and she worked diligently on the tasks presented.

Results of the *WISC-R* indicate overall average range cognitive functioning with verbal expressive skills somewhat lower than psychomotor but not significantly. No true weaknesses were noted in the testing. Michelle appears to have average range command of the English language. She has gained an age-appropriate amount of information from experiences and education, practical knowledge and social judgment, ability to manipulate number concepts, verbal concept formation, and ability to define vocabulary. A relative weakness was noted in auditory memory and sequencing.

Psychomotor skills appear to be at the upper limits of the average range in ability to recognize essential details, visual-motor perception and coordination, and relationships of parts to whole. A relative weakness, though within the average range, was noted in ability to learn unfamiliar tasks.

In summary, Michelle's overall cognitive functioning is within the average range with average range verbal skills and psychomotor skills at the upper limits of the average range. No true weaknesses were noted.

School Psychologist

Psycho-Educational Evaluation

Tests Administered

Malcomesius Screening Test

Visual Memory	*88%*
Visual Discrimination	*100%*
Visual Memory/Written Response	*77%*
Auditory Memory/Written Response	*81%*

Woodcock-Johnson Psycho-Educational Battery: Tests of Cognitive Ability

Visual Perceptual Speed	GE *8.8*	AE *14-2*	%ile *47*	SS *99*
Visual Matching (100%)		Grade Range *6.0–8.0*		
Spatial Relations (88% items/73% puzzles)		Grade Range *12.9*		
Auditory Memory	GE *5.4*	AE *10-8*	%ile *19*	SS *87*
Memory for Sentences		Grade Range *1.5–3.0*		
Numbers Reversed		Grade Range *5.0–8.0*		

Wide Range Achievement Test-Revised: Spelling

GE *5.2* %ile *7* SS *78*

Woodcock-Johnson Psycho-Educational Battery: Tests of Achievement

Reading	GE *5.1*	AE *10-4*	%ile *17*	SS *86*

Word Identification		Grade Range *8.0–10.0*		
Word Attack		Grade Range *2.0–3.0*		
Passage Comprehension		Grade Range *4.0–5.0*		
Mathematics	GE *7.0*	AE *12-4*	%ile *21*	SS *88*
Calculation		Grade Range *8.0–9.0*		
Applied Problems		Grade Range *5.0–7.0*		
Written Expression	GE *7.4*	AE *12-10*	%ile *32*	SS *93*

Test of Written Language: Written Language Quotient *82*

Vocabulary	%ile *9*	SS *80*
Thematic Maturity	%ile *16*	SS *85*
Word Usage	%ile *16*	SS *85*
Style	%ile *9*	SS *80*

Classroom Reading Inventory (Silvaroli) Listening Comprehension

Level	Comprehension
4th grade	*80%*
5th grade	*70% (Instructional level)*
6th grade	*60%*
7th grade	*40%*

Testing Interpretation

Learning Modality. On the *Malcomesius,* Michelle demonstrated adequate visual memory skills, however, she made two "b-d" reversals. On the visual discrimination of words task she scored 100%. Visual memory with a written response appears to be an area of difficulty. On the spatial relations task she focused on the parts rather than the whole. She experienced difficulty with all visual sequencing of numbers tasks and made two transpositions of letters errors. On the abbreviated auditory memory to written test, Michelle did well on the sequencing of words, but experienced difficulty with sequencing numbers.

On the *Woodcock-Johnson,* Michelle's performance on the Visual Perceptual Speed tasks was appropriate for age, grade, and cognitive expectations. On the visual matching of numbers at the 6.0–8.0 grade range, she correctly responded to all items attempted. On the spatial relations subtest, her score of 12.9 grade range appears to be more a reflection of speed than accuracy at 88% accuracy on items and 73% accuracy on puzzles.

Michelle's overall performance on the Auditory Memory Cluster was nearly 3½ years below expectation for age and grade functioning. Memory for sentences at 1.5–3.0 grade range appears somewhat depressed due to one word substitution errors on three tasks that retained the sentence meaning. Michelle experienced difficulty with the numbers reversed task, which was also noted on the *WISC–R* Digit Span and *Malcomesius* number sequencing.

Reading and Listening Comprehension. Michelle's performance on the *Woodcock-Johnson* indicates reading functioning at the 5.1 GE or almost four years deficit for age and grade expectancy. On the word identification subtest, she scored above expectancy at the 8.0–10.0 grade range. A significant weakness was noted in word attack skills at the 2.0–3.0 grade range. Michelle appeared to look at the first letter of the nonsense words and guess. Phonics and structural analysis skills do not appear well enough developed to be of much use in decoding unfamiliar words. Passage comprehension appears a significant weakness by 3–4 years at the 4.0–5.0 grade range.

Listening Comprehension appears to be a significant weakness for Michelle. On the *Silvaroli,* her instructional level was 4th–5th grade range, similar to her reading comprehension. At the higher levels she experienced significant difficulties with inference, cause-effect, and evaluation questions. She correctly responded to vocabulary definition and literal level questions.

Written Expression. On the *Woodcock-Johnson,* Michelle scored about 1½ years deficit for grade expectancy in mechanics of written expression. Her primary area of difficulty was in spelling. She demonstrated adequate skills in the area of proofing: determining correct spelling, punctuation, and word usage. Spelling appears to be a significant weakness at nearly 4 years deficit for grade expectations on the *WRAT-R.* Michelle experienced difficulty with phonetic spellings, single and double vowels, omission of syllables. She refused to continue the spelling test after she missed 8 out of 10 words.

On the *TOWL,* Michelle scored significantly below expectations in word usage, capitalization, and punctuation in isolation. Her thematic maturity (story structure) and use of higher level vocabulary in her written language sample were significant weaknesses. Informal assessment of her written sample indicated a very immature story for age and grade expectancy. She described the pictures rather than writing an integrated story with beginning, middle, and ending. She wrote in run-on sentences not using her knowledge of capitalization and punctuation.

Mathematics. Michelle's overall performance in mathematics at the 7.4 GE indicates 1½ years deficit for grade expectations. Calculation at 8.0–9.0 grade range is within grade expectancy. She experienced difficulty with fractions and could not remember how to reduce or change the answer to a mixed number. Michelle's performance on applied problems is significantly weaker than calculation at 5.0–7.0 grade range. She understands two-step problems. She experienced difficulty with problems dealing with percentages, measurement, fractions, money, and pounds.

Summary. Michelle appears to have specific visual and auditory skill deficits rather than one learning channel substantially weaker than the other. She experienced difficulty with tasks requiring visual memory with a written response, auditory sequencing of numbers, and auditory memory of words.

Michelle is functioning below age, grade, and cognitive expectancy in all academic areas. She functions at grade level in areas in which skills are learned by rote including word identification and calculation. All areas requiring application of skills or reasoning including listening comprehension, passage comprehension, applied problems, written expression are difficult for Michelle. Processing problems in visual memory with a written response and auditory memory appear to significantly impact her abilities to learn phonics and other word attack skills which negatively impacts spelling ability.

Educational Diagnostician

Social and Emotional Development (Informal Assessment)

Michelle is making progress in social and emotional development. She has attended small-group sessions which met twice per week for 30 minutes all school year focusing on social and emotional development areas.

Social Perspective-Taking. Michelle's social perspective-taking abilities have increased in recognition and showing concern about how others feel and in expressing concern for others. She makes inferences about the characteristics of people, but has difficulty in anticipating how another's personality will affect her own behavior (social inferences). She is developing more insight into the reciprocal nature of social interactions and is developing the ability to observe herself and others and engage in social comparison.

Social Regulation and Moral Development. Michelle conforms to several sets of rules regarding moral codes and behaviors (e.g., family, church, peers). She functions basically at a literal level so experiences difficulty with the nuances of written and unwritten rules and codes of conduct. She does not learn easily through indirect socialization methods. Michelle has improved in regulating her own behavior according to social rules and is able to participate in more rule-governed games without loosing self-control when she does not win. She understands that appropriate behavior differs in various social settings, but may break the rules when with a group of friends (e.g., giggling in church or in the library). Michelle is sensitive to the negative reactions of others and is very upset regarding her academic failure.

Social Problem-Solving. Michelle experiences difficulty in the area of social problem-solving skills. Since she experiences difficulty with cause and effect relationships in academic areas, it is not surprising to see that she also experiences difficulty in social areas. Michelle functions primarily on a literal level, she does not always perceive the social consequences of her behaviors.

Social Relationships: Peers. Michelle interacts with peers in unsupervised social situations, but most of her peer interactions are supervised either formally or informally. She dresses according to appropriate standards of her peer group. She primarily "hangs out" with several girls that she has known since primary grades. Moving to a new home will not necessitate changing friends as she will attend the same school and church. She is very sensitive to the feelings of her best friends. Michelle is not allowed to date until she is 16 years old and is not very sophisticated concerning dating relationships. She is eager to attend high school in the fall and various dances and co-ed activities.

Summary. Michelle experiences difficulty with social inferences, social problem-solving, cause-effect relationships, and social consequences of various behaviors. She is fairly typical for an 8th grade girl, perhaps a little immature.

Guidance Counselor

Vocational Assessment

Tests Administered

Informal Leisure Inventory	*Satisfactory*
Informal Vocational Interest Survey	*Child Day Care Specialist*
Work Behaviors Simulations	*Satisfactory*
Daily Living Skills Simulations	*Satisfactory*
Informal Social Skills Survey	*Adequate*
Competitive Employment Survival Skills	*Adequate*

Testing Interpretation

Daily Living Skills. Michelle's previous academic assessment indicates that she possesses the basic mathematics skills to learn to compute family finances, create a simple budget, and balance a checkbook. Her reading skills are high enough to learn to follow recipes and essentials of meal planning. Michelle cares for her own basic personal needs. She demonstrated adequate skills in food preparation and clothing care. Michelle assists with food preparation, house-keeping, laundry, ironing, simple sewing tasks, and yardwork at home. Michelle knows how to drive the lawn tractor, and change the oil in a car. Leisure is spent with her two best friends, and at the activities of the church youth group and the youth organizations to which she and her friends belong.

Personal Social Skills. Michelle appears to possess a fairly stable self-concept. She possesses most of the basic social skills of her social groups.

Occupational Skills. Michelle is a diploma track student who plans to attend the community college after high school graduation and earn an Associate in Applied Science degree in Early Child Development. She plans to work for her aunt in her aunt's Day Care Center, and later own and operate her own small day care facility for preschool children. Currently, she babysits after school. During the summer Michelle works for her aunt, so she is gaining many occupational skills that she will need. Michelle demonstrated 100% of the basic skill requirements of competitive employment.

Academics. Currently, Michelle is a diploma track student.

Vocational Teacher

Evaluation Summary

Michelle is a 14 year old student just completing the eighth grade. Cognitively, she is functioning within the average range with average range verbal expressive skills and psychomotor skills at the upper limits of the average range. No true weaknesses were noted.

Learning modality deficits appear to be interfering with academic functioning. She experiences difficulty with tasks requiring visual memory with a written response, auditory sequencing, and auditory memory.

Academically, Michelle is functioning below age, grade, and cognitive functioning in all academic areas. She functions at grade level in skills areas that can be learned by rote such as word identification (8.0–10.0 grade range) and calculation (8.0–9.0 grade range). She functions below expectancy in areas requiring application of skills and reasoning such as reading comprehension (4.0–5.0 grade range), applied problems (5.0–7.0 grade range), written expression (approximately 5th grade level), and listening comprehension (4th–5th grade level). Visual and auditory processing difficulties significantly interfere with learning phonics and spelling skills. Study skills (e.g., note taking during lectures) are significantly hampered by problems in auditory memory and listening comprehension.

Social development appears to be somewhat immature. Michelle experiences difficulty with social inferences, social problem-solving, cause-effect relationships, and social consequences.

Michelle is a diploma-track student. Her vocational assessment indicates no specific concerns. At this point she does not plan to be a part of the Work-Study Program.

Case Manager

DIAGNOSIS: Learning Disabled (listening comprehension, basic reading skills, reading comprehension, math reasoning, written expression)

Chapter Seven

CASES OF PHYSICALLY AND OTHER HEALTH IMPAIRED STUDENTS

"Physically and other health impaired students include a very heterogeneous population including orthopedically and neurologically impaired children.... The intellectual abilities of physically and other health impaired children and youth range from severe/profound retardation to gifted; therefore, a generalized statement about cognitive or academic learning problems of these children cannot be made" (Jones, 1992, 149). Physical impairments include congenital conditions (e.g., clubfoot) and conditions caused by diseases (e.g., poliomyelitis). Neurological impairments such as cerebral palsy and spina bifida are caused by damage to the central nervous system. Chronic health problems include asthma, sickle cell anemia, cardiac disorders, cystic fibrosis, and AIDS.

Preschool Age/Grade: See Mark & Jeff
Primary Age/Grade: April
Intermediate Age/Grade: See Erica & Heather
Secondary Age/Grade: Wesley
(See also Randy)

RE-EVALUATION REPORT
APRIL

Age: 7 years, 8 months
Grade: 2nd Grade
Date: April , 19___

Background and Educational Concerns

Reason for Referral

April is a 7 year, 8 months old student attending a special day school for physically handicapped students. She has attended this school since she was three years old. April has spina bifida and was shunted in infancy for hydrocephalus. She has made enormous progress in physical therapy and self-help skills. This special re-evaluation was requested because April's teachers feel that she could successfully be mainstreamed to the public schools. In the past parents have been opposed to mainstreaming because April has made significant progress with intensive physical therapy in the special day school.

Health

School records indicate that April's immunizations are current. A physical examination several months ago indicated no specific concerns.

Medical records indicate a diagnosis of spina bifida (myelomeningocele) accompanied by paralysis and loss of sensation in the lower trunk and lower limbs, and loss of bowel and bladder control. As an infant she was shunted for hydrocephalus and experiences none of the typical characteristics. She walks with crutches and braces to support her legs and trunk.

Vision and Hearing Screenings

School screenings indicate normal range visual and auditory acuities.

Speech and Language Screenings

Speech screening indicated articulation, voice, and fluency were within normal limits. Language screening indicated adequate pragmatics, syntax, and semantics. April experienced significant difficulty with morphology including verb tenses, plurals, and comparatives.

Behavior History

Teachers report that April is a very conscientious student, highly motivated, and very task oriented. She is a very friendly little girl who wants to do things for herself. She enjoys being around other children and has a sunny disposition.

Socio-Economic and Home Information

English is the language of the home. April is the oldest of three children of a bank president and his second wife. Her preschool-aged brothers are nonhandicapped. The children appear to get along well together. Parents have been very concerned about April's handicapping condition and have sought professional assistance since her infancy. They have spared no expenses on hiring private physical therapists and purchasing equipment at home to match that at school. Mother has been very involved in carrying out the home programming. The family lives in an affluent neighborhood and has their own swimming pool. April takes piano, drawing, and swimming lessons; brothers take gymnastics and swimming.

MULTIDISCIPLINARY EVALUATION

This evaluation includes the following assessments: intelligence, academic achievement, motor, and social skills.

Psychological Evaluation

Test Administered

Wechsler Intelligence Scale for Children-Revised (WISC-R)

Verbal IQ	*110*	Performance IQ	*112*	Full Scale IQ	*112*
Information	*12*	Picture Completion	*12*		
Similarities	*11*	Picture Arrangement	*13*		
Arithmetic	*10*	Block Design	*12*		
Vocabulary	*14*	Object Assembly	*12*		
Comprehension	*13*	Coding	*10*		
Digit Span	*12*				

Testing Interpretation

April is a 7 year, 8 months old, second grade student who has spina bifida. She came to the testing situation in a friendly and out-going manner. Rapport was readily established and she appeared highly motivated.

Results of the *WISC-R* indicate that overall cognitive abilities fall within the high average range with little variability among verbal expressive and psychomotor abilities. No true weaknesses were noted in her performance. Relative strengths were noted in vocabulary knowledge and judgment in social situations. Relative weakness was noted in ability to manipulate number concepts.

There were no true strengths or weaknesses among psychomotor skills. Relative strength was noted in nonverbal judgment, social alertness, and common sense. Relative weakness was noted in speed of visual-motor reaction and association of symbols.

In summary, April's performance on the *WISC-R* indicates intellectual functioning within the high average range with little variability among verbal expressive and psychomotor abilities, and no true strengths or weaknesses.

School Psychologist

Psycho-Educational Evaluation

Tests Administered

Slingerland Screening Test, Form B

Far Point Copying	*Good*
Near Point Copying	*Good*
Visual Discrimination	*100%*
Visual Memory	*98%*
Visual Memory/Written Response	*92% sequencing/94% items*
Auditory Memory/Written Response	*88% sequencing/90% items*

Diagnostic Achievement Battery (DAB)

Listening	Quotient *103*		
Story Comprehension		%ile *50*	SS *10*
Characteristics		%ile *63*	SS *11*

Speaking	Quotient *97*		
Synonyms		%ile *91*	SS *14*
Grammatic Completion		%ile *5*	SS *5*
Reading	Quotient *124*		
A/Word-Knowledge		%ile *99*	SS *17*
Reading Comprehension		%ile *63*	SS *11*
Writing	Quotient *120*		
Capitalization		%ile *37*	SS *9*
Punctuation		%ile *84*	SS *13*
Spelling		%ile *98*	SS *16*
Written Vocabulary		%ile *91*	SS *14*
Mathematics	Quotient *103*		
Math Reasoning		%ile *63*	SS *11*
Math Calculation		%ile *50*	SS *10*
Spoken Language	Quotient *100*		
Written Language	Quotient *123*		

Testing Interpretation

Learning Modality. April's performance on the *Slingerland* indicates average range functioning for age and grade expectations. Auditory and visual learning channels appear adequate with an oral or a written response. There appears to be no significant learning modality deficits.

Reading and Listening. April's overall performance on the *DAB* in reading indicates very superior functioning for age, grade, and cognitive functioning. A significant strength is her superior range word recognition ability. She demonstrated superior range phonics and structural analysis skills. April used her superior word attack skills in decoding unfamiliar words. Performance in reading comprehension appears average for age, grade, and cognitive expectations. She responded correctly to detail, main idea, and inference questions.

April's listening skills appear to be adequate for age, grade, and cognitive expectations. She functioned within the average range in both story comprehension and characteristics. She correctly responded to detail, main idea, vocabulary, inference, and sequencing questions after listening to a story. On the characteristics test, April interpreted sentences requiring knowledge of the characteristics of objects or events and their various categories.

Speaking. April's overall performance in speaking was adequate for age and grade expectations, but below average for cognitive expectations. On the synonyms test she scored above average for cognitive expectations. The synonym test assessed both receptive and expressive language abilities, primarily semantics. Performance on the grammatic completion subtest was significantly deficit for age, grade, and cognitive expectations. Her functioning indicates a significant deficit in morphology including plurals, possessives, verb tenses, comparative and superlative adjectives.

Writing. April's performance in writing indicates above-average functioning in writing for age, grade, and cognitive expectations. Her ability to capitalize skeleton sentences was in the average range, while punctuation was in the above-average range. April's performance in spelling was in the superior range. On the written expression sample, April's use of higher level vocabulary was in the above-average range. She used dialogue in her story but did not always use the quotation marks correctly. Her story was short but included a beginning, middle, and ending; and included action.

Mathematics. April's performance in math calculation and reasoning were in the average range for age and grade expectations. On the calculation test, April correctly calculated 3 and 4 digit numbers with 2 and 3 addends without regrouping and subtracted double digit numbers with no regrouping. She experienced difficulty with renaming, and could not answer any of the multiplication and division basic fact problems. On the math reasoning test, April correctly responded to abstract questions dealing with time to the nearest half hour, simple fractions, identifying basic monetary coins (e.g., nickel, dime, quarter), and responded correctly to problems requiring addition or subtraction; and two-step problems.

Summary. April appears to have good visual and auditory learning abilities with an oral or written response. She appears to be functioning academically within the average to superior range in all academic areas. Average-range spoken language is significantly weaker than superior range written language. The only subtest with less than average range functioning was grammatical completion which was quite poor indicating a significant weakness in the morphological aspects of language.

Educational Diagnostician

Motor and Self-Help Evaluation (Informal Assessment)

April is an enthusiastic student, a quick learner, who has a great desire to be independent in school and self-help tasks. Due to spina bifida, there are a number of concerns or potential problems that teachers, therapists, and April must be alert to including: (1) Symptoms of shunt blockage, (2) Symptoms of urinary infections/problems, (3) Symptoms of skin breakdown, (4) Prevention of deformities, and (5) Psycho-social problems.

Gross Motor Skills. April ambulates using braces and crutches or a swivel walker. She is making good progress in gait training and independence in mobility. April needs continued assistance in mobility skills including handling stairs and getting on and off the school bus independently. She, also, requires some assistance in checking braces and skin to avoid problems. She requires some modifications in her physical education program in activities involving running and jumping.

Due to spina bifida, April lacks sensation to touch, pressure, pain and temperature (anesthetic skin) in lower extremities which can lead to breakdown of skin on buttocks and under braces. To avoid skin break down and joint deformities in spine, hips, and legs, she must change positions frequently. A standing frame, various positioning alternatives, and periods of sitting alternated with periods of activity are helpful. Since April is so academically task focused, she may need to be reminded to vary positions and activities. A timer is often helpful.

Fine Motor Skills. April is completely age appropriate and independent in fine motor skills. Her handwriting is neat and legible.

Self-Help Skills: Eating. April is completely independent (age appropriate) in eating skills. Bowel and bladder control require that she maintain consistent eating and drinking patterns and amounts. In the school cafeteria, she will need someone to carry her tray to the table and should be allowed an end or corner seat so she will not have to climb over benches.

Self-Help Skills: Toileting. Toileting is a major concern for independence and mainstreaming. April has completed bowel training, scheduling elimination at home. For urination, she is independent in self-catheterization every 3 hours. She may feel more secure performing this task in the bathroom adjacent to the nurse's office in case of problems.

Self-Help Skills: Dressing. April is independent in dressing. She often wears wide legged slacks that can fit over braces or wears dresses with matching bloomers. Putting on rainboots is a problem, but she is independent in putting on most outdoor apparel.

Physical Therapist

Social and Emotional Skills Evaluation (Informal Assessment)

April is a delightful 2nd grade student who gets along well with her peers and teachers at the special school. Most of the physically impaired students in her class have lower intellectual abilities, so she is accustomed to being the best student, academically, in the class. She has a perfectionist streak about her academic work in terms of neatness and accuracy. In small classes she has been the recipient of frequent praise and appears to thrive on it. She is very sensitive to criticism, mistakes, and teasing.

Social Perspective-Taking. April engages in social perspective-taking, as she recognizes and shows concern for others in her class and at the special school. She is very sensitive to pain and illness that others may experience. She has great concern for children who cannot walk at all.

Due to parents concern for development of social skills, social communication and appropriate behavior in numerous social settings have been significantly stressed at home and at school. April understands that different behaviors are called for in various school settings (e.g., library, the classroom, recess), and in various home and community settings (e.g., dinner guests, church, children's theatre, playroom). She understands how to greet persons and initiate conversation, and to take-turns in conversation. April interacts with some nonhandicapped peers regularly in her social activities. Since she is the only handicapped child in most of these settings, she is often pampered and waited on.

The success of April's transition to the public school classroom from the special school environment may well lie with the social-emotional issues in peer interactions such as the following: (1) Maintenance and increasing April's independence, (2) Dealing with not being the best student in everything, (3) Peers' reactions to her handicapping conditions. Thus, April's class will need transitioning training for appropriate peer interactions and encouraging April's independence.

Guidance Counselor

Evaluation Summary

April is a 7 year, 8 months old student attending a special day school for physically handicapped students. Cognitively, April is functioning within the high average range with little variability among her psychomotor abilities and verbal expressive skills. She has good visual and auditory perceptual and motor integration skills.

Academically, April is functioning within the average to superior range for age, grade, and cognitive expectations in all academic areas. The only true weakness is in the language area of grammatical completion or the morphological aspects of language in which she is functioning severely deficit for age, grade, and cognitive expectations.

Motor skills assessment indicates that April's fine motor skills are age appropriate. Gross motor skills are severely deficit due to spina bifida. She walks with leg braces and crutches. Due to anesthetic skin she needs to change positions frequently; a standing frame is helpful. April needs an adapted physical education program. She experiences difficulty independently handling stairs and getting off and on the school bus.

Most self-help skills are independent. Eating skills are age-appropriate. Toileting has been controlled this past year through bowel training and scheduling elimination at home; and self-catheterization every 3 hours for urination control. She knows the signs and symptoms of shunt blockage, urinary infections, and skin breakdowns.

Though socially a delightful, friendly well-adjusted student in the special day school, there are concerns regarding her successful transition to the public school classroom in terms of maintaining her independence and motivation, fostering appropriate interactions with nonhandicapped peers, and self-acceptance and self-expectations in academics.

Case Manager

DIAGNOSIS: Physically Impaired (Spina Bifida)

RE-EVALUATION REPORT
WESLEY

Age: 13 years, 10 months
Grade: 8th grade
Date: May   , 19____

Background and Educational Concerns

Reason for Referral

Wesley is a 13 year, 10 months old 8th grade student functioning in the bottom third of his 8th grade class. His current diagnosis is Other Health Impaired due to severe asthma and severe allergies. Last September he had one half lung surgically removed due to mold infestation. He received Home Bound services in September and October and returned to school in November.

Current concerns include academic functioning and study behavior. Academically, Wesley failed most of his 1st semester classes. During the second semester he was placed in a special program for lower functioning Junior High students. He is not successful in this program. Wesley has a very short attention span and frequently "drifts off." He seldom completes and hands in homework. He does not appear to understand that the homework grades count as one-third of his overall class grade.

The purpose of this special re-evaluation is to determine appropriate placement and programming for the next academic year.

Health

Immunizations are current. Wesley has severe asthma and allergies (e.g., mold, plant pollens, dust; foods with nuts, soy, and wheat products). Last September one half of his left lung was surgically removed due to severe mold spore growth. Wesley takes significant amounts of medication (injections and orally) especially during the spring and fall. He is extremely allergic to bee stings, and many foods especially those containing nuts, soy, or wheat. He carries an antidote kit and there is one in the nurse's office in case of emergencies. Accidental ingestion of foods with nuts, soy, or wheat cause his throat to swell shut—the result could be suffocation. Once the adrenalin from the emergency kit is injected, he has 20 minutes to get to the hospital.

Wesley carries a special breathing atomizer to clear his airway when he is experiencing breathing difficulties. He takes medication morning and evening at home.

Wesley brings his lunch to school due to his special diet. He takes adapted physical education classes. Going up long flights of stairs at school are difficult during high allergy stress periods. Wesley often misses a significant amount of school during the spring and fall, and is quite susceptible to bronchitis and pneumonia. (Medical records are in school health file.)

Vision and Hearing Screenings: Normal Range Acuities

Speech and Language Screenings: Within Normal Limits

Behavior

Wesley appears to have no significant behavioral problems. He interacts appropriately with adults and peers. Teachers indicate that he experiences significant difficulty with sustained attention and his attention span is very short. Usually he does not get angry when teachers attempt to refocus him.

Socio-Economic and Home Information

English is the language of the home. Wesley, his younger sister Sarah, and parents live in a settled neighborhood of small thirty-year old split level brick homes. His father is an automobile mechanic who has numerous old cars in and near the garage that he is fixing for people after work. Mother works as a checker in the local grocery store.

At home Wesley has regular chores including taking out the trash and keeping his room straightened. He helps with the cooking, especially preparation of his special diet foods. There appear to be no major home concerns regarding behavior. Wesley observes family curfew. He is pitcher on the neighborhood softball team, but most of his exercise is from swimming. He has several friends that have been buddies since primary grades and hangs out with them. There appears to be no economic deprivation.

CURRENT MULTIDISCIPLINARY EVALUATION

This evaluation includes assessments in the areas of intelligence, perception and memory, academic achievement, and vocational skills.

Psychological Evaluation

Test Administered

Wechsler Intelligence Scale for Children-Revised (WISC-R)

Verbal IQ	*84*	Performance IQ	*96*	Full Scale IQ	*89*
Information	*6*	Picture Completion	*10*		
Similarities	*8*	Picture Arrangement	*10*		
Arithmetic	*8*	Block Design	*7*		
Vocabulary	*8*	Object Assembly	*12*		
Comprehension	*7*	Coding	*9*		
Digit Span	*7*				

Testing Interpretation

Wesley is a 13 year, 10 months old 8th grade student. He entered the test setting somewhat apprehensively, but once begun he was friendly, appropriate, and attended well to the numerous short tasks with good effort.

Results of the *WISC-R* indicate overall cognitive abilities within the upper limits of low average intellectual functioning with borderline verbal expressive skills and average range psychomotor skills. Verbal expressive skills in practical knowledge and social judgment, auditory memory and the ability to manipulate number concepts, verbal concept formation, language vocabulary knowledge, and attention and auditory sequencing skills are within the average to low average range. Weakness was noted in Wesley's fund of information gained from experience and education.

Psychomotor abilities reveal a wide range of skills from high average to low average functioning. A significant strength is noted in visual-motor coordination and assembly skills. Visual alertness to details and nonverbal judgment using picture clues represents average range functioning. Wesley performed in the lower limits of the low average range in analysis and reproduction of abstract designs and in speed of ability to learn symbols and shapes and to recreate them.

In summary, Wesley's overall cognitive functioning is within the low average range with borderline verbal skills and average psychomotor skills. Verbal expressive weaknesses were noted in his fund of information and in understanding appropriate behaviors in various social settings.

School Psychologist

Psycho-Educational Evaluation

Tests Administered

Malcomesius Screening Test

Visual Memory/Written Response	*88% items/100% sequencing*
Auditory Memory/Written Response	*88% items/90% sequencing*

Woodcock-Johnson Psycho-Educational Battery: Tests of Cognitive Ability

Visual Perceptual Speed Cluster	GE *11.4*	AE *18-2*	%ile *73*	SS *104*
Visual Matching (96%)				Grade Range *10.0–12.9*
Spatial Relationships (76% items/58% puzzles)				Grade Range *5.0–8.0*
Auditory Memory Cluster	GE *6.9*	AE *12-4*	%ile *16*	SS *85*
Memory for Sentences				Grade Range *3.0–6.0*
Numbers Reversed				Grade Range *5.0–8.0*

Woodcock-Johnson Psycho-Educational Battery: Tests of Achievement

Reading		GE *8.2*	AE *13-4*	%ile *43*	SS *97*
	Word Identification	Grade Range *6.0–9.0*			
	Word Attack	Grade Range *7.0–12.9*			
	Passage Comprehension	Grade Range *9.0–11.0*			
	Synonyms-Antonyms	Grade Range *6.0–9.0*			
	Analogies	Grade Range *5.0–7.0*			
Mathematics		GE *5.6*	AE *11-0*	%ile *9*	SS *80*
	Quantitative Concepts	Grade Range *8.0–11.0*			
	Calculation	Grade Range *5.0–7.0*			
	Applied Problems	Grade Range *5.0–7.0*			

Wide Range Achievement Test-Revised: Spelling

GE *5.4* %ile *14* SS *84*

Test of Written Language: Written Language Quotient *83*

Vocabulary	%ile *25*	SS *90*
Thematic Maturity	%ile *16*	SS *85*
Word Usage	%ile *16*	SS *85*
Style	%ile *25*	SS *90*

Classroom Reading Inventory (Silvaroli)

Level 7	Listening Comprehension *80%*
Level 8	Listening Comprehension *60%*

Testing Interpretation

Learning Modality. Wesley's overall performance on the *Malcomesius* and *Woodcock-Johnson* indicate that the visual channel is a good learning modality for him. He has good visual memory with a choice or written response. Visual sequencing of letters and words, and visual discrimination of numbers are areas of strength. Wesley experienced difficulties in the area of spatial relationships in both speed and accuracy.

Wesley's overall performance on the *Malcomesius* and the *Woodcock-Johnson,* also, indicate that the auditory channel is a good learning modality for him. On a test of short-term memory for sentences, Wesley performed in the severe deficit range primarily due to adjective substitution that did not change the meaning of the sentences. On an informal test of auditory memory with a written response, Wesley performed within expectations. Auditory sequencing and reorganization of numbers appears to be a strength.

Reading and Listening Comprehension. Wesley's performance in reading on the *Woodcock-Johnson* indicates average functioning for age, grade, and cognitive expectations. Primary areas of weakness include word identification (grade range 6.0–9.0), synonyms and antonyms (grade range 6.0–9.0), and analogies (grade range 5.0–7.0). Wesley's oral reading was fluent. He used his knowledge of phonics and syllabication skills in decoding unfamiliar words. He utilized context clues effectively in decoding unfamiliar words and in deriving meaning. Passage comprehension at Grade Range 9.0–11.0 is an area of strength. Reading appears to be an area of strength for Wesley. He indicated that oral reading helps him to concentrate.

Wesley's performance in listening comprehension on the *Silvaroli* indicates low average functioning for age and grade expectations. At the

7th grade level he scored 80% on comprehension questions, and 60% at the 8th grade level. He experienced difficulty with questions requiring definition of vocabulary, a weakness previously noted in vocabulary comprehension (e.g., synonyms, antonyms, analogies).

Written Expression. Wesley's overall functioning in written expression indicates low average functioning for age and grade expectations, but commensurate with his verbal intelligence scores. In spelling on the *WRAT-R,* Wesley appeared to be relying primarily on his good visual memory skills. He experienced difficulty with polysyllabic words, primarily on the middle syllables. He needs to apply his knowledge of word attack skills to spelling.

On the *TOWL* Word Usage subtest, Wesley's performance was below age and grade expectations, but commensurate with cognitive expectations. His primary areas of weakness included verb tenses and pronoun antecedents. His performance on the Style subtest (capitalization and punctuation) revealed average functioning for age and grade expectations. Areas of weakness included correctly using the following punctuation marks: apostrophes, commas, quotation marks, and commas.

Wesley's use of higher level vocabulary words in his expressive writing sample was in the average range. He utilized eleven higher level vocabulary words. He did, however, appear to experience difficulty using precise words and proper nouns to convey ideas. His performance on the Thematic Maturity subtest (story content and structure) was below age and grade expectations, but commensurate with cognitive expectations. He experienced difficulty with remembering the facts of his story and caused confusion by relating conflicting details (e.g., "the planet Earth blew up and the earthlings returned home").

Informal assessment of the written language sample indicated that Wesley did not write in complete sentences. He did not utilize his knowledge of capitalization and punctuation. He did not write an integrated story due to lack of sequential development. Wesley did not write in paragraphs.

Mathematics. Wesley's overall performance in mathematics indicates functioning in the deficit range for age, grade, and cognitive expectations. Primary areas of deficit include both calculation and applied problems (Grade Range 5.0–7.0). He appears to understand the algorithms of addition, subtraction, single digit multiplication, and simple division. He appears to know the basic facts in addition, subtraction, multiplication, and division. Wesley experienced difficulty with the process of double-digit multiplication. He attempted, unsuccessfully, to compute double digit long division problems in his head. He indicated that he had forgotten how to change improper fractions to mixed numbers.

On the applied problems subtest, Wesley's performance revealed good abstract (mental) calculation skills. He demonstrated strengths in abstract reasoning ability. He revealed understanding of relationship concepts that indicate which mathematical process is required in problem solving. Wesley, however, revealed a lack of understanding of computation of two-step problems. He demonstrated strengths in calculating problems dealing with money, but weaknesses in computing time and measurement. His performance revealed difficulties in sorting through extraneous information to isolate basic information required to solve problems. Significant strengths were displayed in the area of quantitative concepts (grade range 8.0–11.0). Wesley preferred to estimate an answer rather than do the computations.

Summary. Wesley appears to experience learning modality deficits in the area of spatial relationships. Both visual and auditory channels are adequate for learning with an oral or written response. Academically, reading is an area of strength for Wesley. Mathematics, both calculation and applied problems, appear to be areas of significant weakness. Though written expression skills in isolation appear adequate, Wesley experienced significant difficulty utilizing them in the construction of a written product. He also experienced significant difficulty writing complete sentences and paragraphs.

Educational Diagnostician

Vocational Evaluation

Tests Administered

Informal Leisure Inventory	*Satisfactory*
Informal Vocational Interest Survey	*Auto Mechanic*
Work Behaviors Simulations	*Satisfactory*
Daily Living Simulations	*Satisfactory*
Personal Social Skills	*Satisfactory*
Informal Social Skills Survey	*Satisfactory*
Occupational Skill Level Survey	*Apprentice Level*

Test Interpretation

Daily Living Skills. Wesley's performance indicates that he possesses basic mathematics skills, especially if he uses a calculator, to compute family finances and create a simple budget. He possesses basic home maintenance skills such as cleaning house and washing dishes. He demonstrates skills in food preparation (special diet) and clothing care, but he needs more experiences in mending and ironing. Wesley cares for his own personal needs as showering, shaving, etc. without reminders. Leisure time is spent in participating in sports, watching sports on TV, and hanging around the shop.

Personal Social Skills. Wesley appears to possess a fairly stable self-concept. Within his socio-economic environment, he possesses basic social skills. He does need some assistance in social communication skills and in social problem-solving skills as he functions better nonverbally. Generally, personal social skills is an area of strength for Wesley.

Occupational Skills. While occupational decisions are tentative pending health, Wesley generally plans to attend auto mechanic school and work with his father in his mechanic shop. He possesses a great deal of practical experience, "apprenticing" with his father since middle grades. During work simulations he demonstrated skills in general auto maintenance (e.g., changing oil and filters).

Academic Skills. Wesley has a definite strength in the area of reading. He experiences deficits in multiplication and division in mathematics. He has some basic written expression skills, but needs to focus on writing sentences and paragraphs. Lack of study skills, motivation, and attention deficits in combination with frequent absences due to asthma and allergies severely impact his academic progress. Wesley is failing most of his academic areas because he does not complete homework, does not know how to prepare and write papers, and has very poor organization skills.

Vocational Teacher

Evaluation Summary

Wesley's overall cognitive functioning is within the low average range with borderline verbal skills and average psychomotor skills. His verbal weaknesses were in his background fund of knowledge and in social problem solving. Psychomotor weaknesses primarily involved spatial relationships. Both visual and auditory learning modalities appeared adequate.

Academically, reading (GE 8.2) appears to be an area of strength for Wesley. Mathematics (GE 5.6), both calculation and applied problems, appear to be areas of deficit for cognitive expectations. Wesley, also, experiences deficits in written expression for grade level expectancy. His deficits in attention, organization, and study skills impact all areas. An initial vocational evaluation indicated that Wesley is making satisfactory progress in daily living skills, personal-social skills, and occupational skills.

Wesley currently has a diagnosis of Other Health Impaired due to severe asthma and allergies, but he is not receiving any specific academic services unless he needs HomeBound services. Last September he had one-half of his left lung surgically removed and missed the first few months of school. He receives adapted physical education. Wesley is on a special diet brought from home to avoid nuts, soy, and wheat. He carries an antidote kit for severe allergy reactions, and one is kept in the school nurse's office. He often misses large blocks of time from school during the fall and spring.

Case Manager

DIAGNOSIS: Other Health Impaired

Chapter Eight

CASES OF GIFTED AND TALENTED STUDENTS

Renzulli (1986) emphasizes that the gifted individual must demonstrate productivity and that research on creative/productive people has consistently shown that although no single criterion should be used to identify giftedness, persons who have achieved recognition because of their unique accomplishments and creative contributions possess a relatively well-defined set of three interlocking clusters of traits: above average ability, task commitment, and creativity.

It is not the superior ability but the interaction between these traits or clusters of traits which contribute to giftedness (Renzulli, 1978).

Preschool Age/Grade: See Cara
Primary Age/Grade: Cory
Intermediate Age Grade: See Erica & Nicole
Secondary Age/Grade: See Daniel

EVALUATION REPORT
CORY

Age: 6 years, 11 months
Grade: 1.8
Date: May , 19___

Background and Educational Concerns

Reason for Referral

Cory is a 6 year, 11 months old first grade student at Jackson Elementary School. Cory is an excellent student academically, functioning above expectations within the classroom; a class leader; highly motivated and energetic. She began reading prior to entrance in kindergarten. Cory is also an exceptional artist. During free time she writes and illustrates her own stories that are above age and grade expectations. She is a "whiz" on the computer. Cory was referred for testing by her classroom teacher for consideration for the Gifted Enrichment Program.

Health

Immunizations are current. There are no significant medical concerns.

Vision and Hearing Screenings: Normal Range Acuities.

Speech and Language Screenings: Within Normal Limits

Socio-Economic and Home Information

Cory is the daughter of a primary grade teacher (mother) and the County Attorney (father). She has an older brother, Roy, who is in the 3rd grade. The family lives in a small town in a three-story 100-year-old restored Colonial Williamsburg home. The parents completed much of the restoration and often spend free time at estate sales and antique shops where they have accumulated most of the furnishings for the home. Cory and Roy are the only grandchildren on both sides of the family. There is no social or economic deprivation.

CURRENT MULTIDISCIPLINARY EVALUATION

This evaluation includes assessments in intelligence, perception and memory, academic achievement, and abilities and interests.

Psychological Evaluation

Tests Administered

Wechsler Intelligence Scale for Children-Revised (WISC–R)

Verbal IQ	*135*	Performance IQ	*130*	Full Scale IQ	*132*
Information	*17*	Picture Completion	*16*		
Vocabulary	*17*	Picture Arrangement	*17*		
Arithmetic	*16*	Block Design	*16*		
Similarities	*17*	Object Assembly	*15*		
Comprehension	*17*	Coding	*16*		
Digit Span	*17*				

Testing Interpretation

Cory is a 6 year, 11 months old 1st grade student who entered the testing situation eager to participate. She was friendly and well-behaved and worked diligently throughout the testing period. She was verbally spontaneous and showed great facility with language and with social conversational skills for her age.

Results of the *WISC–R* indicate overall gifted range functioning (lower limits) with no significant differences among verbal expressive and psychomotor abilities. Cory demonstrated gifted verbal expressive abilities for age expectations in information gained from experience and education, in the use of complex and abstract language, in abstract verbal concept formation, in the use of social judgment, and in auditory memory and sequencing ability. There were no verbal expressive weaknesses.

Cory's overall psychomotor skills fall within the lower limits of the gifted range. There were no true weaknesses. She demonstrated strength in visual alertness to detail and organization, in nonverbal judgment and common sense, in analysis and reproduction of abstract designs, in visual-motor coordination, and in speed of visual-motor reaction and association of symbols.

In summary, Cory is a very pleasant, verbally spontaneous first grade student whose overall cognitive functioning is within the lower limits of the gifted range with no significant weaknesses.

School Psychologist

Psycho-Educational Evaluation

Tests Administered

Slingerland Screening Test Form B (2nd and 3rd grade)

Far-Point Copying	*Good*
Near-Point Copying	*Good*
Visual Memory	*100%*
Visual Discrimination	*88%*
Visual Memory/Written Response	*93% items/100% sequencing*
Auditory Memory/Written Response	*100% items/100% sequencing*
Auditory Discrimination	*94%*
Auditory Visual Association	*100%*

Woodcock Reading Mastery Tests (Form A)

Word Identification	GE *3.5*	%ile *98*	SS *131*
Word Attack	GE *5.8*	%ile *98*	SS *131*
Word Comprehension	GE *2.9*	%ile *87*	SS *117*
Passage Comprehension	GE *3.1*	%ile *92*	SS *121*
Total Reading	GE *3.8*	%ile *99*	SS *135*

Informal Written Expression Test

Capitalization	Grade 2
Punctuation	Grade 2
Vocabulary	Grade 2
Word Usage	Grade 2

Test of Written Language

Spelling	%ile *75*	SS *110*
Word Usage	%ile *75*	SS *110*
Style	%ile *37*	SS *95*

Formal Reading Inventory (FRI)

Listening Comprehension	%ile *98*	Quotient *132*
Levels:		Comprehension:
1st grade		*80%*
2nd grade		*70%*
3rd grade		*80%*
4th grade		*80%*
5th grade		*60%*
6th grade		*60%*

Key Math Diagnostic Arithmetic Test GE *3.2*

Calculation		Applied Problems	
Addition	GE *2.4*	Numeration	GE *3.8*
Subtraction	GE *2.7*	Fractions	GE *3.8*
Multiplication	GE *3.9*	Geometry	GE *2.4*
Division	GE *2.4*	Mental Computation	GE *4.4*
		Numerical Reasoning	GE *4.4*
		Word Problems	GE *3.2*
		Missing Elements	GE *3.9*
		Money	GE *2.5*
		Measurement	GE *3.1*
		Time	GE *3.0*

Testing Interpretation

Learning Modality. Cory's overall functioning on the *Slingerland* indicated above-average functioning for age and grade expectations. Both visual and auditory channels with oral or written response appear strong ways of learning for Cory. Visual memory of words, letters, and numbers appears excellent. On the visual discrimination task she experienced a "b-d" reversal, and on the visual memory with a written response she reversed a "3." All letter, number, and word sequences were accurate.

Reading and Listening Comprehension. Cory's performance on the *Woodcock* indicates functioning at GE 3.8, significantly above age and grade expectations. Word identification (GE 3.5) and word attack (GE 5.8) are areas of significant strength. Word comprehension (GE 2.9) and passage comprehension (GE 3.1) are somewhat weaker, but above age and grade expectations for a 1st grade student. Cory's oral reading is fluent, effectively using phonics, syllabication, and context clues in decoding unfamiliar words.

Listening comprehension at the 4th grade instructional level is an area of significant strength. Cory functioned nearly at instructional level at the 6th grade level. She experienced some difficulty with vocabulary definition questions at the higher levels. Cory answered the inference, detail, main idea, and cause-effect questions with accuracy. She utilized context clues to gain meaning.

Written Expression. On the *Slingerland,* Cory's near-point and far-point copying exercises revealed adequate, but hastily formed manuscript letters. She experienced difficulty with uniformity of size and spacing of letters and words. On the *TOWL,* she experienced significant difficulty with near-point copying of sentences, sometimes writing an entire sentence with no spacing between words. Her creative writing was legible but spacing and size were still areas of difficulty.

Cory was administered three subtests of the *TOWL,* Spelling and Word Usage indicated above-average functioning for age expectations, while Style (capitalization and punctuation) was in the average range. Analyzation of the spelling test indicated excellent functioning in spelling phonetic words, but difficulty with spelling nonphonetic words. On the Word Usage task, Cory experienced difficulty with verb tenses. Strengths were evident in forming comparatives and regular plurals. The Style subtest indicated difficulty in capitalizing proper nouns (names, months, countries). Her basic skills included capitalizing the first word of the sentence and using a period or question mark at the end.

The spontaneous creative writing sample indicated above-average functioning for grade level. She wrote in complete sentences (13 sentences), beginning with a capital letter and ending with a period. The story had a specific beginning "Once upon a time" and a definite conclusion. It involved a social problem and eventual resolution to the problem. Cory experienced a number of spelling errors in the written sample.

Mathematics. Cory's overall functioning on the Key Math (GE 3.2) indicated significantly above-average functioning for age and grade expectations. In addition, Cory can add several digit numbers with no regrouping. She appears not to understand the concept of regrouping (e.g., carrying). In subtraction, Cory subtracted correctly double digit numbers with no regrouping. On the multiplication subtest, Cory demonstrated her knowledge of some basic facts (e.g., 8×3). She was able to answer several picture questions involving division, but no basic fact questions.

Cory's individual subtests in applied problems generally indicates significant strength compared to calculation abilities. Mental computation and numerical reasoning (GE 4.4), missing elements (GE 3.9), numeration and fractions (GE 3.8) are significant areas of strength. Though, relative weaknesses were shown in geometry and symbols, word problems, money, measurement and time, these areas are at least 6 months to one year above grade expectations.

Summary. Cory's performance indicates visual and auditory channels with oral or written response are good ways of learning. She did not appear to experience any significant perceptual processing deficits. Academically, Cory is functioning significantly above age and grade expectations in all subjects.

Abilities and Talents (Informal Assessment)

Artistic Ability

Cory produces exceptional art products for age and grade expectations. She is very good at pencil drawing reproductions of items she sees. She frequently illustrates stories that she has written. Last summer, Cory participated in art enrichment activities including making pottery, water color painting, wire sculpture, and paper mache. She shows a definite eye for line, form, symmetry, design, and color. Due to her interest in art, parents have an art center at home for her use. Parents indicate that she is always creating something.

Dramatic Ability

Cory participates in after school drama club. She has shown great facility in memorizing lines and in extemporizing when peers have forgotten their lines. She has helped to plan plays including characters, plot, scenery, and costumes. She shows great facility with language.

Computer Skills

Cory is a "whiz" on the computer. She often uses word processing in writing her stories. She can, also, use graphics to illustrate the stories. She can play many computer games, and completes academic programs designed for much older students.

Violin Ability

Cory has taken violin lessons since she was 3 years old. She enjoys lessons and practicing at home, as well in performing with the children's orchestra. She plays very well for age expectations.

Literature

Cory is a voracious reader, reading a wide variety of books both fiction and nonfiction. She often completes an art project depicting an aspect of the books that she reads. She often models stories that she writes on stories read.

Foreign Language

Cory is studying German with lessons once each week. Her family toured Germany last summer and plan another trip next year. She has shown an amazing facility and interest in languages.

General Abilities and Interests

Cory appears interested in a wide range of topics and fields. Her parents have a well-stocked library and activity room for Cory and her brother. She has very good visual planning and organization skills, good eye-hand coordination, and completes many projects quickly and creatively while peers are still deciding what to do. She is very good at occupying herself during free periods, however, she usually does not go on to a new project until the current one is completed. She moves rapidly from one activity to another, is self motivated in task completion, and is very concerned regarding accuracy and/or quality. Academically she has been allowed to progress as rapidly as she wishes, independently completing assignments and taking skills tests.

Gifted Facilitator

Evaluation Summary

Cory is a 6 year, 11 months old 1st grade student. Results of the WISC–R indicate overall gifted range functioning (lower limits) with no significant differences among verbal expressive and psychomotor skills. Both auditory and visual channels appear to be excellent modalities for learning.

Academically, Cory appears to be functioning in excess of two years above age and grade expectations in reading, listening comprehension, and mathematics. Her handwriting revealed hastily formed letters and problems with uniform spacing and size. Performance in written expression mechanics and composition is above-average for age and grade expectations. Currently, she is programmed individually in most academic areas.

Cory appears interested and talented in many areas including art, music, drama, and languages. She has excellent motivation and good organizational skills, and good task focus and completion skills. She is a classroom leader. Cory is friendly and well-liked among peers and teachers.

Case Manager

DIAGNOSIS: Gifted and Talented

BIBLIOGRAPHY

Alpern, G., Boll, T. & Shearer, M.: *Developmental Profile II.* Aspen, CO: Psychological Development Publications, 1980.

Bayley, N.: *Bayley Scales of Infant Development.* New York: Psychological Corp., 1969.

Beery, K. & Buktenica, N.: *Developmental Tests of Visual-Motor Integration.* Chicago: Follett, 1982.

Brigance, A.: *Brigance Inventory of Basic Skills.* North Billerica, MA: Curriculum Associates, 1977.

Brigance, A.: *Brigance Diagnostic Inventory of Early Development.* North Billerica, MA: Curriculum Associates, 1978.

Boehm, A.: *Boehm Test of Basic Concepts-Revised.* Cleveland, OH: Psychological Corp., 1985.

Cattell, P.: *Cattell Infant Intelligence Scale.* New York: Psychological Corp., 1960.

Davis, C.: *Perkins-Binet Tests of Intelligence for the Blind.* Watertown, MA: Perkins School for the Blind, 1980.

Deckert, L., McCartney, J. & Podleski, J.: *Social Communication Skills for Handicapped Adolescents.* Town & Country, MO: Special School District of St. Louis CO, 1989.

Dunn, L. & Dunn, L.: *Peabody Picture Vocabulary Test-Revised.* Circle Pines, MN: American Guidance Service, 1981.

Durrell, D. & Catterson, J.: *Durrell Analysis of Reading Difficulty* (3rd ed.). San Antonio, TX: Psychological Corporation, 1980.

Federal Register: *Implementation of Part B of the Education of the Handicapped Act.* Washington, DC: U.S. Government Printing Office. (42478), August 23, 1977.

Frankenburg, W., Dodds, J., Fandal, A., Kazuk, E., Cohrs, M.: *Denver Developmental Screening Test-Revised.* Denver, CO: Ladoca Publishing, 1975.

Frost, J.: *Developmental Checklists for 3-, 4-, and 5-Year-Olds.* Austin, TX: University of Texas at Austin, 1972.

Goodenough, S. & Harris, D.: *Goodenough-Harris Drawing Test.* Cleveland, OH: Psychological Corporation, 1963.

Hammill, D. & Larsen, S.: *Test of Written Language.* Austin, TX: pro-ed, 1983.

Hiskey, M.: *Hiskey-Nebraska Test of Learning Aptitude.* Lincoln, NE: Author, 1966.

Jastak, S. & Wilkinson, G.: *Wide Range Achievement Test-Revised.* Wilmington, DE: Jastak Associates, 1984.

Jones, C.J.: *Social and Emotional Development of Exceptional Students: Handicapped and Gifted.* Springfield, IL: Charles C Thomas, 1992.

Kieran, S., Connor, F., Von Hippel, C. & Jones, S.: *Mainstreaming Preschoolers:*

Children with Orthopedic Handicaps. Washington, DC: U.S. Department of Health & Human Services, 1980.

Koppitz, E.: *Bender Visual Motor Gestalt Test.* New York: Grune & Stratton, 1963.

Larsen, S. & Hammill, D.: *Test of Written Spelling-2.* Austin, TX: pro-ed, 1986.

Lee, L.: *Northwest Syntax Screening Test.* Evanston, IL: Western University Press, 1971.

Leiter, R. & Arthur, G.: *Leiter International Performance Scale.* Chicago: Stoelting, 1980.

Lesiak, W.: *Developmental Tasks for Kindergarten Readiness.* Brandon, VT: Clinical Psychology, 1978.

Lillie, D. & Harbin, G.: *Carolina Developmental Profile.* Winston-Salem, NC: Kaplan School Supply, 1975.

Malcomesius, N.: *Specific Language Disability Test: Grades Six, Seven, and Eight.* Cambridge, MA: Educators Publishing Service, 1967.

Markwardt, F.: *Peabody Individual Achievement Test-Revised (PIAT-R).* Circle Pines, MN: American Guidance Service, 1989.

McCarney, S., Leigh, J. & Cornbleet, J.: *Behavior Evaluation Scale.* Columbia, MO: Educational Services, 1983.

Newborg, J., Stock, J., Wnek, L., Guidubaldi, J. & Suinicki, J.: *Battelle Developmental Inventory.* Allen, TX: DLM Teaching Resources, 1984.

Nihira, K., Foster, R., Shellhaas, M. & Leland, H.: *AAMD Adaptive Behavior Scale.* Washington, DC: American Association for Mental Deficiency, 1974.

Reid, D., Hresko, W., & Hammill, D.: *Test of Early Reading Ability.* Austin, TX: pro-ed, 1981.

Silvaroli, N.: *Classroom Reading Inventory* (5th ed.). Dubuque, IA: Brown, 1986.

Slingerland, B.: *Pre-Reading Screening Procedures to Identify First Grade Academic Needs.* Cambridge, MA: Educators Publishing Service, 1977.

Slingerland, B.: *Slingerland Screening Tests for Identifying Children with Specific Language Disability.* Cambridge, MA: Educators Publishing Service, 1970.

Sparrow, S., Balla, D. & Cicchetti, D.: *Vineland Adaptive Behavior Scales.* Circle Pines, MN: American Guidance Service, 1984.

Stillman, R. (Ed.): *The Callier-Azusa Scale.* Dallas: Callier Center for Communication Disorders, University of Texas at Dallas, 1978.

Swanson, H. & Watson, B.: Speech Development (p. 140–141). *Educational and Psychological Assessment of Exceptional Children* (2nd ed.). Columbus, OH: Merrill, 1989.

The Conover CO.: *Survival Skills System.* Omro, WI: Author, 1990.

Thorndike, R., Hagen, E. & Sattler, J.: *Stanford-Binet Intelligence Scale* (4th ed.). Boston, MA: Houghton-Mifflin, 1986.

Wechsler, D.: *Weschler Adult Intelligence Scale* (WAIS). New York: The Psychological Corporation, 1974.

Wechsler, D.: *Wechsler Intelligence Scale for Children-Revised.* New York: The Psychological Corporation, 1974.

Wechsler, D.: *Wechsler Preschool and Primary Scale of Intelligence* (WPPSI). New York: The Psychological Corporation, 1974.

Weiner, J.: Classroom Demands Interview Record Form, Interview Questions on Essay/Project/Report Writing, Checklist for Assessing Student's Examinations, Checklist for Assessing Student's Notebook, Gaining Information from Text. In Alternatives in the Assessment of the Learning Disabled Adolescent: A Learning Strategies Approach. *Learning Disabilities Focus,* 1 (2), 97–107, 1986.

Wepman, J.: *The Auditory Discrimination Test.* Palm Springs, CA: Language Research Associates, 1975.

Woodcock, R. & Johnson, M.: *Woodcock-Johnson Psycho-Educational Battery: Tests of Cognitive Ability-Revised.* Allen, TX: DLM Teaching Resources, 1989.

Woodcock, R. & Johnson, M.: *Woodcock-Johnson Psycho-Educational Battery: Tests of Achievement.* Allen, TX: DLM Teaching Resources, 1989.